Carb Cycling Cookbook for Beginners
© Copyright 2024 by Merry Lott

Remember to speak with your doctor before starting any new diet, especially if you have any underlying health conditions or nutritional concerns. While restrictive low-carb or high carb diets may not be suitable for everyone.

First Edition: May 2024

Cover: Illustration made by Merry Lott

TABLE OF CONTENTS

CHAPTER 1
INTRODUCTION TO CARB CYCLING

What is Carb Cycling?

Carb cycling is a nutritional strategy that involves purposefully varying your carbohydrate intake from day to day. Rather than constantly eating a regular or moderate amount of carbs daily, you cycle between low-carb days and high-carb days. This intelligent approach to carbs aims to help optimize fat loss and muscle growth.

On low-carb days, your carbohydrate intake is restricted to put your body into a state of ketosis. Ketosis occurs when your liver begins converting fat into fatty acids and ketone bodies to be used for fuel, rather than relying primarily on glucose from carbs. Being in ketosis promotes tapping into stored body fat for energy, enabling you to burn fat more efficiently. However, very low carb intake for too many days consecutively can sometimes impede performance and muscle growth.

Therefore, the high-carb days in a carb cycling plan serve to replenish glycogen stores (glucose energy stored in the muscles and liver). Glycogen is the body's preferred immediate fuel source for intense workouts and strength training. Periodically increasing your carbohydrate consumption can boost gym performance, power, and endurance while also aiding muscle repair and growth.

The strategic cycling of low-carb and high-carb days offers the benefits of ketosis without the drawbacks of staying ultra-low-carb for too long. Carb cycling provides just enough carbohydrate intake to support your workouts and fuel your muscles adequately. Yet you still reap the accelerated fat-burning effects during a sufficient number of low-carb days.

Typically, carb cycling involves eating 20-50 grams of net carbs for 1-3 days consecutively, followed by 1-2 days of increased carb intake of around 150-200 grams. However, the optimal carb cycling ratio depends on your gender, body composition goals, activity levels, and personal carb tolerance.

For females, a general recommendation is to consume about 30-50 grams of carbs on low-carb days and 120-150 grams on high days. Males can usually handle slightly higher carb intakes of 50-150 grams on low days and 200-300 grams on high days. Extended low-carb stints of 4 or more days are not recommended without medical supervision.

On the low-carb days, you will get carbs mostly from fibrous vegetables, some nuts and seeds, as well as a moderate amount of dairy. High-carb days include all the vegetables, dairy, nuts, and seeds, plus the strategic addition of starchy carbohydrates like potatoes, rice, quinoa, beans, or fruit.

It is crucial to time the high-carb days around your most intense or prolonged workout sessions for the week. Increased carbohydrates are used to fuel your workouts and aid in muscle recovery. You may opt to have 1-2 back-to-back high-carb days if you have intense workouts on consecutive days. Or you can separate the high days with clusters of low days in between.

Carb cycling can fit into various styles of eating, like Paleo, Mediterranean, or flexible dieting. It simply involves strategically rotating your carb sources and amounts in a structured, cyclical fashion. You still emphasize whole, unprocessed foods the majority of the time.

Carb cycling requires diligent meal planning and preparation to execute correctly. You need to carefully plan out the days, target carb amounts, and weigh or measure your foods. Tracking apps can help monitor your daily macronutrients. Meal prepping your carb-cycling snacks and meals for the week also saves time.

Be prepared for some possible initial side effects as your body adapts to the low-carb days, like fatigue, headaches, or cravings. Staying well hydrated, consuming enough calories overall, and getting sufficient rest will help minimize adverse effects. It can take a few weeks to become fully fat-adapted.

With consistency using the carb cycling strategy, most people report feeling increased energy, fewer cravings, improved body composition and gym performance. Carb cycling can be continued long term and adjusted as needed over time to keep making progress.

Remember to speak with your doctor before starting any new diet, especially if you have any underlying health conditions or nutritional concerns. While restrictive low-carb diets may not be suitable for everyone, strategic carb cycling offers flexibility. Find what works best for your body through trial and error.

Benefits of Carb Cycling

Carb cycling provides a strategic approach to nutrition that can offer many benefits compared to just winging your carb intake day-to-day or sticking to a moderate carb diet indefinitely. The purposeful cycling between low-carb and high-carb intake days can help optimize body composition, workout performance, hormone balance, and overall health.

One of the primary benefits of carb cycling is enhancing fat loss. Periods of very low carb intake induce ketosis, where your body taps into stored fat for fuel. Ketosis prompts accelerated fat burning, especially from stubborn body fat stores around the midsection and hips. Consuming carbohydrates causes an insulin response, which can inhibit fat burning to some degree. So having frequent periods of low-carb eating coupled with high protein intake provides an excellent metabolic environment for utilizing fat as energy.

In addition, carb cycling can help maintain and build muscle mass. On low-carb days, you are able to burn off excess body fat without sacrificing lean muscle tissue. The ketosis state helps preserve muscle. Then the targeted high-carb days provide your body with adequate glycogen to power through intense workouts and fuel muscle growth. This glycogen replenishment supports athletic performance and aids workout recovery. The result is fat loss paired with muscle gain, and strength increases over time.

Another benefit is the appetite suppressing aspect of being in ketosis during the low-carb phases. Keeping insulin levels low and tapping into fat for fuel can help reduce hunger and cravings. You may find it effortless to go many hours without eating or feeling famished on low-carb days. This makes it easier to maintain a calorie deficit without constant hunger. Furthermore, you may experience boosted energy, focus, and mental clarity once you become fat adapted.

Due to the varying calorie and carbohydrate intake, your body does not adapt to a set point. The calorie cycling can help rev up your metabolism, unlike standard dieting, which often causes adaptive thermogenesis and plateauing. The more extreme carb fluctuation keeps your body responding and continually burning calories. In this way, carb cycling helps overcome weight loss stalls.

Additionally, carb cycling can regulate hormones related to fat storage, stress, and reproductive health. Insulin remains low on most days, which optimizes fat burning hormones. Cortisol levels even out over the week, which reduces belly fat storage related to high stress. For females, carb cycling can help minimize estrogen dominance, regulate the menstrual cycle, and improve conditions like PCOS. Balancing blood sugar is beneficial for fertility and libido as well.

Another advantage of carb cycling is that it is very flexible and customizable. You can tweak the number of low-carb days versus high-carb days and adjust your exact carb grams based on your unique body and needs. The macro percentages can be personalized to your goals, whether they are strictly fat loss, gaining mass, or athletic performance. Carb cycling is compatible with many different styles of eating and can be adapted long-term as your goals change.

Implementing carb cycling does require diligent meal planning and preparation. You need to be organized, motivated, and consistent to reap the rewards. Meal prepping your cyclical diet for the week requires effort. Tracking your macros precisely using a food journaling app is also advised. The rigid schedule and paying close attention to carb intake is not a casual endeavor. However, the carb cycling strategy prevents mindless or emotional eating since every meal and day has a purpose.

In the beginning, there may be some adaptation symptoms during the ultra-low-carb days. Headaches, fatigue, cravings, constipation, or insomnia are common initially before becoming fat adapted. Staying hydrated, getting sufficient sleep, managing stress, and being patient will help you push through the temporary downsides. Within a few weeks, any negative side effects typically resolve.

At first glance, carb cycling may seem unnecessarily complicated. However, once you get into the groove of alternating low-carb and high-carb days, it feels much easier and intuitive. The diligent planning and tracking does require effort.

How Carb Cycling Affects Your Body

Carb cycling creates noticeable effects throughout the body due to the varying levels of carbohydrates consumed from day to day. The metabolic, hormonal, and physiological impacts reflect this nutritional fluctuation. Understanding how your body responds can help you use carb cycling more effectively.

On low-carb days, carb restriction to under 50 grams daily prompts the liver to produce ketones for fuel instead of relying on glucose from carbs. Entering into ketosis activates fat burning, especially from stubborn subcutaneous body fat like belly, hip, and thigh fat. Using fat for energy can enhance mental clarity, stabilize energy levels, and reduce appetite. However, very low carb intake for too long can lead to fatigue, nausea, or decreased athletic performance.

When carb intake is substantially increased on high days, your muscles soak up the glycogen for immediate energy. Stored glycogen provides an accessible power source for intense exercise. Replenishing glycogen aids muscle repair and growth. High-carb days also boost levels of anabolic hormones like insulin, testosterone, and IGF-1, further supporting hypertrophy.

Additionally, high-carb days elicit an insulin response, which helps shuttle amino acids into the muscles along with the glucose. This can accelerate recovery from strength training sessions. However, the heightened insulin levels also instruct your body to start storing fat again instead of burning it. Finding the ideal balance of low and high-carb days allows you to maximize fat loss while still building muscle.

Beyond impacts to energy, metabolism, and hormones, carb cycling can affect other biological functions. For example, digestion speeds up on high carb days. The extra fiber from starchy carbohydrates combined with more calories overall enhances gastrointestinal motility. Healthy bowel movements are common when carb and calorie intake increases.

However, some people experience digestive issues like constipation, bloating, or diarrhea during the very low carb days. Removing fiber from grains and most fruits and veggies can slow things down. Consuming probiotic foods helps counteract this. Drinking plenty of fluids is also key to staying regular when carb intake is very low.

Carb cycling causes obvious fluctuations on the scale weight due to glycogen storage changes. Glycogen bonds with water molecules in the body, so high-carb intake increases water retention. Low carb intake depletes glycogen and results in water loss. It is common to drop several pounds in the first week due to this diuretic effect. The scale weight spikes back up on high-carb days as glycogen and water replenish.

For females, carb cycling can help regulate reproductive hormones and the menstrual cycle. Extended periods of low-carb intake may trigger changes in estrogen, progesterone, cortisol, and thyroid hormones. Some women experience changes to their period, cycle length, or related symptoms when significantly reducing carb intake. The higher carb days can help counterbalance hormone fluctuations.

Mental outlook and sleep quality may also be impacted by carb cycling. Low-carb days tend to improve focus and mood in most people initially. However, very low carb intake for too long can backfire and cause irritability, anxiety, or insomnia in some people. The higher carb days boost serotonin production, which usually enhances mood and sleep. Finding the right balance is key.

In summary, carb cycling noticeably impacts fat burning capabilities, muscle building potential, energy levels, digestion, hormones, and more. Tracking your stats and symptoms provides insight into how your body responds best. Be aware of both the benefits and drawbacks of low and high-carb days. Develop a customized carb cycling plan that optimizes your own physiology and goals. Remaining flexible and observant will enable you to reap the full benefits.

Setting Realistic Goals

When embarking on a new carb cycling diet, it is crucial to set clear and achievable goals for yourself. Having realistic expectations helps keep you motivated over the long run. Outlining both short-term and long-term benchmarks enables you to chart your progress and celebrate successes.

A comprehensive goal-setting process is recommended when starting a carb cycling plan. First, reflect on your current situation, including your weight, body composition, fitness level, health, and lifestyle factors. Consider any issues you want to improve or conditions needing management. Assess your schedule, responsibilities, and potential barriers like social events or work travel.

Then envision your ideal objectives in both the near and distant future. Common goals for carb cycling may include losing fat, gaining muscle, boosting fitness, normalizing blood sugar, improving cholesterol, regulating hormones, reducing inflammation, or alleviating digestive issues. Defining your motivations and required outcomes drives the goal setting process.

With your targets defined, break them down into smaller, quantifiable steps to make the process less intimidating. Set specific weekly and monthly milestones that gradually move you towards your end goals. Outline the tangible actions required to hit each marker. Goals should be realistic yet challenging enough to feel rewarding when achieved.

A recommended technique is setting SMART goals for your carb cycling diet:

- **Specific** - zero in on exact desired outcomes, like losing 1 pound per week or gaining 5 pounds of muscle mass within 3 months. Vague goals are hard to accurately work towards.

- **Measurable** - frame goals in quantitative terms you can track like clothing size, body measurements, body fat percentage, macros tracked, workout performance metrics, lab tests, etc.

- **Achievable** - challenge yourself, but set goals you can realistically accomplish with consistency. Consider your schedule, environment, and physical limitations.

- **Relevant** - your goals must align with the purpose of carb cycling for optimal body composition, fitness, or health. Ensure they address your needs.

- **Time bound** - attach specific time frames to each goal, like losing X pounds per week or gaining X amount of strength in X months. This creates accountability.

Here are some examples of effective SMART goals for a carb cycling diet:

- "Lose 1 pound per week for the next 3 months by adhering to the prescribed low and high carb days."

- "Increase my bench press by 20 pounds within 2 months through dedicated strength training 4 times per week."

- "Decrease body fat percentage from 25% to 20% in 6 months through carb cycling and HIIT workouts."

- "Lower A1C from 6.2 to below 5.7 within 6 months by following my custom carb cycling plan consistently."

Tracking apps, body measurements, before photos, and performance benchmarks make it easy to quantify progress towards your defined goals. However, the scale weight will fluctuate dramatically due to carb cycling. Do not rely solely on scale weight to measure fat loss. Take weekly progress photos and measurements of your waist, hips, chest, thighs, and arms instead. The visual changes in the mirror better show body recomposition.

Adapt your workouts, nutrition tracking rigor, and meal plans over time based on results. Make note of what is working well for your body and what may need tweaking. Be prepared to adjust your goals if they were set too conservatively or aggressively. Life circumstances can also impact your trajectory. The most sustainable approach is to aim for slow and steady progress over quick fixes.

Remember that slip-ups are inevitable. Expect occasional backslides, and do not let one indulgence derail your motivation. Simply restart the very next day. Even top athletes, models, and bodybuilders incorporate planned cheat periods into their regimented diets. Strategically designed refeeds or high-carb days prevent metabolic slowdown and burnout.

Share your goals with a support system and ask for accountability. Having cheerleaders and people to check in regarding your benchmark timing, nutrition, and workouts amplifies success. Consider hiring a coach, trainer, or nutritionist for extra oversight and motivation. Surrounding yourself with positive social influences curbs isolation and discouragement.

With SMART goal setting, tracking quantifiable metrics, adaptability, and support, you can transform your body composition one small win at a time through carb cycling. Celebrate each mini-victory to build confidence and momentum. Stay consistent with your plan and believe in your ability to realize ambitious yet realistic fitness goals.

Merry Lott

CHAPTER 2
FUNDAMENTALS OF NUTRITION

Understanding Carbohydrates, Proteins, and Fats

Carbohydrates, proteins, and fats are the three primary macronutrients that provide our bodies with energy and are the building blocks for cell structure and function. Knowing which food sources contain each is fundamental to implementing an effective carb cycling plan.

Carbohydrates include starches, sugars, and fiber. They largely get broken down into blood glucose (sugar), which the body preferentially burns for quick energy. Good sources of whole, unprocessed carbs are whole grains like oats, brown rice, and quinoa; starchy vegetables like sweet potatoes and squashes; beans and legumes; and fruits. These contain important vitamins, minerals, antioxidants, and fiber. Simple or refined carbs like white bread, candy, sugary drinks, and most packaged snacks provide fast energy but lack overall nutrition.

On low carb days of the cycle, you restrict even whole carb sources. Fibrous green vegetables, seeds, nuts, and moderate dairy provide what little carbs you need each day. On higher carb days, you strategically reintroduce whole grain starches, starchy vegetables, and some fruits while still avoiding added or refined sugars. Depending on your calorie needs and activity output, carb intake on higher days ranges from around 75-150 grams for women or 100-300+ grams for men.

Protein provides the building blocks for maintaining, repairing, and rebuilding muscle tissue. Without adequate protein from food sources, you eventually break down muscle mass. Protein also helps you feel full and satisfied after eating. Lean animal proteins, including chicken, turkey, fish, eggs, Greek yogurt, cottage cheese, protein powders; beans, lentils, and soy foods; nuts and seeds are all great options. You need around 0.6-0.8 grams of protein per pound of body weight daily as a baseline, and more if highly active.

Protein intake remains consistent every day of the carb cycling plan because your muscles require it no matter how your carb or fat intake fluctuates. Consuming protein at each meal stabilizes blood sugar when carb intake is lowered on some days. Adequate protein enables you to lose pure body fat without sacrificing lean muscle mass when in a calorie deficit. Many carbcyclers even increase protein slightly on lower carb days for satiety.

Healthy fats provide long lasting energy, help absorb vitamins, support detoxification, regulate cholesterol and blood sugar, decrease inflammation, and aid in fat burning. Excellent sources are oily fish, avocados, olive oil, nuts and seeds, coconut oil, full fat dairy, eggs, and dark chocolate. Limit fried and highly processed fats from fast food, crackers, chips, donuts, etc.

On low carb days, dietary fat intake is usually substantially increased to provide energy and fuel ketosis in the absence of many carbs. You may consume 50-70% of your total calories from healthy fats when carb intake is very low during the cycle. Good fat sources to increase are coconut oil, avocados, olives, and olive oil, nuts, nut butter, full fat dairy like cheese, fatty fish like salmon, and eggs cooked in olive oil or coconut oil.

Then, on high-carb days, dietary fat intake decreases. You still emphasize good fats for their benefits, but the percentage of total calories from fats goes down to maybe 30-40% on days when you eat more carbs. This ensures carbohydrates provide ample energy for intense workouts on those days, rather than burning fats alone. Finding the optimal balance of fats and carbs daily allows you to maximize the benefits of each based on your training, recovery, and health goals.

The Science Behind Low-Carb and High-Carb Days

Altering carb intake from day to day elicits changes in hormones, enzymes, and metabolic processes that allow the body to efficiently burn fat while maintaining muscle. Low-carb days ignite fat oxidation pathways, while high-carb days replenish glycogen and spur muscle growth. Understanding the contrasting biochemical effects enables strategic cycling for results.

With minimal dietary carbs and glucose, insulin levels plummet. Low insulin signals the release of stored body fat from adipose tissue so it can be burned for energy via beta-oxidation in the liver.

Enzymes like hormone-sensitive lipase increase to enable the mobilization and release of free fatty acids into the bloodstream. Simultaneously, low insulin increases the activity of carnitine palmitoyltransferase-1, which transports the freed fatty acids into the mitochondria of cells to be oxidized for energy. In this manner, very low carb days strongly promote fat breakdown and oxidation.

However, sustained ultra low carb intake hampers athletic performance and work capacity. As liver and muscle glycogen stores deplete from carb restriction, power output dwindles. Glycogen provides rapidly accessible energy for bursts of intense physical exertion.

This is where the intermittent high carb days prove beneficial. They boost muscle glycogen stores, which provide an immediate energy substrate for physical training. Insulin levels elevate sharply in response to increased carb and overall calorie intake on high days. The hormone-sensitive lipase enzyme becomes less active, which slows fat release. But the heightened insulin drives glucose and amino acids into muscles, which aids recovery and protein synthesis.

A key enzyme called glycogen synthase increases on higher carb days, which rapidly synthesizes new glycogen molecules for storage in the liver and skeletal muscles. This replenishes depleted reserves, allowing you to train hard again. The varying metabolic states make both fat loss and muscle gain possible.

However, immediately following the very high carb days, the drastic insulin spike combined with replete glycogen levels instigates a rebound of lipogenesis - the creation and storage of body fat. Glycogen seeks to bond with water in the body as well, resulting in fluid retention.

So the day after high carb intake, it's best to return to the low end of your carb cycling range. This prevents fat regain and utilizes the restored glycogen to fuel activity and workouts. Strategically cycling between low and high prevents metabolic stagnation and optimizes body composition over time.

Certain hormones also fluctuate throughout the week of carb cycling, which profoundly impacts body fat storage and muscle tissue. Insulin drops sharply on low days, while leptin levels typically decline more gradually. With leptin and insulin levels low, fat burning can commence.

Thyroid hormones T3 and T4 may also decrease when carb-restricting. This slows your metabolism, but only temporarily until carbs are reintroduced. Growth hormone and testosterone often increase during ketosis. This anabolic environment preserves lean mass despite fewer calories overall on low days.

Cortisol can fluctuate during carb cycling depending on the magnitude of the deficit and exercise demands. Chronically high cortisol levels encourage belly fat storage, so managing stress levels throughout the week is key.

Then, on the higher-carb day, insulin surges while boosting leptin. Testosterone, IGF-1, and thyroid hormones also rise in response to the influx of carbs and calories. This facilitates maximal workout performance and accelerated recovery. The ideal balance and timing of low and high days regulate appetite, fat storage, and muscle protein synthesis.

In summary, carb cycling provides metabolic flexibility. Low days promote fat oxidation, and high days optimize muscle gain. The influx of carbs and ensuing hormonal environment on high days enhances glycogen replenishment and strength capacity. A cyclical schedule provides metabolic advantages over sustained keto or standard dieting. Timed macronutrient fluctuation allows for fat loss, muscle retention, and improved body composition long term.

Key Vitamins and Minerals for Optimal Health

Adequate intake of vitamins and minerals is essential for overall wellness and to support the beneficial effects of carb cycling. Key micronutrients affect energy levels, metabolism, immunity, workout recovery, and more. When restricting entire food groups during the diet, be proactive about sufficient vitamin and mineral consumption.

Firstly, the B-complex vitamins play numerous roles in converting food into cellular energy. Thiamin (B1), riboflavin (B2), niacin (B3), pantothenic acid (B5), pyridoxine (B6) and cobalamin (B12) all help metabolize fats, proteins, and carbs. Deficiencies in these can cause fatigue. Great sources are poultry, fish, eggs, dairy, beans, nuts, seeds, and leafy greens.

Vitamin B6 benefits amino acid metabolism for muscle protein synthesis. Vitamin B12 is crucial for red blood cell formation, neurological function, and DNA synthesis. Low B12 is common with extended meat and dairy restrictions on very low carb diets. Supplement if necessary.

Vitamin C powerfully reduces inflammation and stimulates collagen formation for wound healing. It also combats exercise-induced oxidative stress. Citrus fruits, red bell peppers, broccoli, strawberries, and tomatoes contain high levels.

Vitamin D supports calcium absorption and bone health, but also impacts immune function, mood, and heart health. Get regular sun exposure, eat fatty fish, and supplement vitamin D3 if deficient. Optimal levels near 50 ng/ml are advised.

Vitamin E protects cell membranes. It acts as an antioxidant to reduce damage from free radicals during exercise. Nuts, seeds, whole grains, spinach, and avocados provide vitamin E.

Vitamin K improves blood clotting and vascular health. The K1 form is abundant in leafy greens like kale, spinach, and swiss chard. Vitamin K2 occurs in dairy, eggs, and fermented foods. K2 specifically helps bones utilize calcium.

Minerals like magnesium, zinc, and calcium also deserve attention. Magnesium aids muscle recovery, sleep quality, blood sugar control, and electrolyte balance. Spinach, almonds, avocados, black beans, and pumpkin seeds are great sources.

Zinc supports immune function, protein synthesis, DNA formation, and wound healing. Oysters, animal proteins, seeds, legumes, and yogurt supply dietary zinc. Over 30% of people are deficient, so supplement if you restrict these foods.

Calcium builds strong bones and teeth while enabling nerve impulse transmission and enzyme function. Dairy products, leafy greens, almonds, and salmon provide calcium. Vitamins D and K2 also facilitate calcium absorption and bone mineral density.

With severe carb restriction, intake of these beneficial micronutrients declines due to eliminating grains, fruits, and energy-dense carbs. Be diligent about including the best sources during all phases of the carb cycling plan. For example, eat ample non-starchy vegetables, nuts, seeds, and lean proteins on low carb days.

On higher carb days, reintroduce sources like starchy tubers, quinoa, fruit, and yogurt. A daily multivitamin can provide nutritional insurance as well. Timed supplementation before or after workouts proves optimal for carb cycling programs.

For instance, take a calcium and vitamin D supplement before training to optimize bone health. After exercise, magnesium, zinc, and anti-inflammatory antioxidants aid recovery and immunity. Case studies demonstrate that adequate micronutrient intake enhances metabolic, body composition, and performance outcomes from carb cycling.

Avoid excessive or prolonged restriction of any food group to prevent potential vitamin and mineral deficiencies. If adhering to extended ketosis diets, special attention must be paid to a sufficient intake of B-vitamins, iron, selenium, phosphorus, and chromium, which aid energy and blood sugar balance. Monitor lab work annually and supplement accordingly.

Work with a registered dietitian or nutritionist to create a custom carb cycling meal plan that meets all your micronutrient needs while accounting for any pre-existing deficiencies or health conditions. Timed supplementation, paired with mindful food choices, makes achieving optimal vitamin and mineral levels realistic throughout the cycling process. This will amplify all the fitness, health, and longevity benefits of intelligently modulating your carb intake.

Hydration and Its Importance in Fitness

Water makes up over 60% of the human body and serves vital functions that impact physical performance and wellness. Maintaining optimal hydration is crucial when carb cycling and exercising. Dehydration degrades endurance, strength, cognitive abilities, mood, and metabolic efficiency.

Water regulates body temperature, flushes waste from cells, transports nutrients, fuels digestion and metabolism, lubricates joints, cushions organs, and facilitates mineral balance. During exercise, increased perspiration and respiration amplify water needs. Fluid losses exceeding 2% of body weight harm exercise capacity and lead to overheating, fatigue, dizziness, cramps, and heat-related illness if severe. Pre-hydrating and sipping fluids during activities are essential.

Thirst itself is not a perfect indicator of hydration status since it may not arise until dehydration exceeds 1% of body weight. The kidneys also conserve water by reducing urine output when dehydrated, delaying the thirst reflex.

So pay attention to the color and volume of urine as a hydration gauge. Pale yellow to clear urine generally indicates adequate hydration. Dark yellow, amber, or scant volumes reflect under-hydration. The first morning urine color can assess baseline status before drinking.

When carb restricting during the diet, hydration needs further increase. Glycogen depletion reduces water storage in muscles and the liver. Ketosis also promotes mild diuresis as ketones and urea flush water from the body. Monitor urine, thirst, and body weight to sufficiently offset losses.

Pre-hydrate in the days and hours leading up to a heavy workout or sporting event when carb cycling. Drink approximately 5 to 10 milliliters per kilogram of body weight 4 hours beforehand.

Rapidly digesting carbs and electrolytes before exercise optimizes hydration and performance. Sports drinks with 2-5% carbohydrates enhance fluid absorption in the small intestine through active glucose transport. Combining water and concentrated carb-electrolyte beverages extends endurance. Rehydrating post-exercise is also imperative - drink to replace at least 150% of sweat losses.

During workouts, match beverage palatability and composition to exercise duration and intensity. For light activity under 60 minutes, plain, cool water suffices. Above 60 minutes of sustained moderate effort, sports drinks become increasingly beneficial. Their carbohydrates provide fuel while promoting fluid absorption.

Electrolytes like sodium and potassium are critical for hydration and muscle function. Sodium enhances thirst, water retention, and circulation volume, while potassium aids cell hydration, nerve transmission, and muscle contractions. Active individuals lose substantial electrolytes in sweat - replenishing them with beverages avoids cramping and fatigue.

Water alone dilutes blood sodium during prolonged exertion, potentially compromising performance. So sports drinks enhance high intensity, endurance, and hot weather training when carb cycling. Tailor your pre, during, and post workout hydration routines to the phase and demands of carb cycling.

On lower-carb days, increased water intake aids metabolism and offsets mild dehydration. Favor unsweetened coffee, tea, water, and zero-calorie electrolyte beverages over high-sugar sports drinks. Limiting carbohydrate drinks prevents disrupting ketosis. Supplemental electrolytes can offset losses.

Then, on higher carb, higher calorie days, sports drinks prove beneficial. The glucose and electrolytes they contain help replenish depleted glycogen stores and enhance hydration. Time these higher-carb drinks around your toughest workouts for optimal energy and recovery.

Hydration monitoring tips:

- Weigh yourself before and after workouts to assess losses. Every pound lost equals 16 ounces of fluid deficit.
- Observe urine color as mentioned.
- Use thirst as a general guide, but don't rely solely on it.
- Include some salty foods/fluids to offset sodium losses through sweat.
- Drink steadily throughout the day, rather than just at meals.
- Avoid caffeine and alcohol, as they have mild diuretic effects.

Adequate hydration complements all phases of an effective carb cycling program - from promoting satiety on keto days to fueling intense training on carb-fueled days. Consistently monitoring and meeting personalized fluid needs enhances fitness and health gains.

Common Nutritional Myths Debunked

Nutrition is filled with myths, trends, and hearsay that can contradict proven science. Learning to separate nutrition facts from fiction helps construct effective health plans like carb cycling. Here are some prevalent misconceptions debunked by current evidence:

- **Myth 1: You should avoid cholesterol from food**: For decades, dietary cholesterol was vilified as allegedly raising blood cholesterol and heart disease risk. However, studies now confirm dietary cholesterol has a minimal impact on blood cholesterol for most people. Exceptions are those with familial hypercholesterolemia. Otherwise, eggs, shrimp, and other cholesterol-rich foods are fine in moderation.
- **Myth 2: Low fat is best for weight loss**: When fat is removed from processed foods, excess sugar is often added back for palatability. This can increase calorie density while reducing satisfaction. Diets high in protein, fiber, and monounsaturated fats often optimize fat loss better than simply cutting total fat intake.
- **Myth 3: Red meat causes cancer**: Headlines claiming red meat is carcinogenic rely on weak epidemiological data. The studies fail to show clear causation. Lean, unprocessed red meat eaten in moderation provides high-quality protein, vitamins, and minerals. Choosing organic and pasture-raised is ideal.
- **Myth 4: "Superfoods" have magical properties**: Many trendy foods are deemed superfoods but lack robust scientific support for the claims. No food group or ingredient alone determines outcomes. A balanced diet with calorie needs matters most, not single so-called superfoods.
- **Myth 5: Carbs are "fattening"**: This myth arose from confusion between simple and complex carbs. While overconsuming sugar, refined grains, and junk foods drive fat gain, whole-food carbohydrate sources, including fruit, beans, and unprocessed grains, are beneficial for health in appropriate portions. Carb cycling capitalizes on their unique benefits. Demonizing all carbs is imprudent.

- **Myth 6: Fasting detoxes your body:** Our kidneys, liver, lungs, and digestive system already eliminate toxins without prolonged fasting. No evidence proves fasting purges toxins or provides unique health benefits if adequate calorie and nutrient intake is maintained through varied, unprocessed whole foods instead.

- **Myth 7: Microwaving kills nutrients:** Microwaves simply heat and cook foods using short waves of radiation. They don't make ingredients radioactive or deplete nutrients substantially more than conventional cooking. Microwaving is a safe, economical food preparation method.

- **Myth 8: You need protein right after training:** The anabolic window for protein is longer than most supplements claim. As long as you eat high-quality protein spaced throughout the day while carb cycling, exact post-workout timing is not critical.

- **Myth 9: Low salt diets reduce risk:** For heart and metabolic health, refined carbohydrates cause far more problems than salt for most individuals. Sea salt provides electrolytes that aid hydration and muscle function without posing health risks in typical amounts.

- **Myth 10: Sugar causes diabetes:** Type 1 diabetes is autoimmune and genetic, unrelated to sugar intake. While obesity and inactivity can greatly increase the risk of preventable type 2 diabetes, sugar alone does not directly cause diabetes. However, excess sugar does promote insulin resistance, weight gain, and other metabolic problems.

By learning the facts, you can optimize nutrition, body composition, and health when carb cycling. Rely on rigorous science to separate truth from hype. Intelligently designed carbohydrate cycling nourishes the body without the need for restrictive diets, miracle foods, or misguided dogma.

CHAPTER 3
EFFECTIVE EXERCISE ROUTINES

Exercises for Low-Carb Days

When carb intake is restricted, glycolytic/anaerobic energy systems become limited. This means high intensity training and heavy weight lifting will suffer during low carb phases. The low fuel state necessitates specific exercise selection on low days - namely fat-burning aerobic workouts. Here are effective routines for low carb days:

- **Low-moderate intensity cardio:** On reduced carbs, stick to zone 2 heart rate training utilizing aerobic energy systems. This burns stored fat more readily without glycogen. Options include easy cycling, incline walking, elliptical training, swimming, and rowing for 45-90 minutes. Heart rate should not exceed 180 minus your age.

- **Circuit training:** Perform successive rounds of bodyweight, plyometric, and resistance training exercises targeting all major muscle groups. The active rest between stations keeps heart rate elevated to sustain fat burning. This builds cardiovascular endurance while preserving lean mass better than straight steady state cardio.

- **HIIT workouts:** Although intensity diminishes on low carb days, brief high-intensity intervals can still elevate metabolism post-exercise. Alternate short 15-60 second bursts of hard work with 1-3 minutes of active rest. This spikes fat burning hormones and enzymes optimally despite low fuel. Options include sprints, bike/rower tabatas, shuttle runs, and kettlebell complexes. Just limit total session duration to 20-30 minutes.

- **Yoga and mobility work:** Low intensity practices focused on joint mobility, balance, flexibility, and mindfulness perfectly suit low energy days. Gentle asanas, stretching, and myofascial release using foam rollers or therapy balls provide activity without taxing glycogen levels. Enhanced mobility aids recovery too.

- **Resistance training:** Lift lighter loads at moderate tempo for higher reps on reduced carbs. Lower intensity prevents premature fatigue but still stimulates muscles. Use shorter rest periods as well. Compound lifts, circuits, lunges, deadlifts, and squats work well. Save heavy barbell exercises for high carb days.

Monitor perceived exertion so you don't overdo activity. Consume some easily digestible carbs about 30 minutes pre-workout on low days to provide minimal glucose for the session. Then refuel after training with protein and fat. Two to three low carb workouts weekly suffices for maintaining fitness and burning stored body fat efficiently.

Exercises for low carb days PRACTICE

On low-carb days, focusing on strength training is beneficial because your body will primarily use fat for fuel. Here, we'll cover exercises targeting all major muscle groups, providing three exercises each. These exercises are designed to help you build muscle and strength efficiently on days when your carb intake is lower.

1. Chest

Bench Press

- Lie back on a flat bench with a barbell.

- Grip the barbell slightly wider than shoulder-width.
- Lower the bar to the middle of your chest.
- Push the bar back up until your arms are fully extended.
- Perform 3 sets of 8-12 repetitions.

Push-Ups

- Start in a plank position with your hands slightly wider than shoulder-width apart.
- Lower your body until your chest nearly touches the ground.
- Push through your palms to lift yourself back to the start.
- Complete 3 sets of 12-15 repetitions.

Dumbbell Flyes

- Lie on a flat bench with a dumbbell in each hand.
- Extend your arms above your chest with a slight bend at the elbows.
- Slowly lower the weights in an arc motion until you feel a stretch in your chest.
- Bring the dumbbells back together using the same arc motion.
- Aim for 3 sets of 10-12 repetitions.

2. Back

Pull-Ups

- Hang from a pull-up bar with an overhand grip.
- Pull yourself up until your chin is above the bar.
- Lower yourself back down to full arm extension.
- Complete 3 sets of as many repetitions as you can.

One-Arm Dumbbell Row

- Place one knee and the same hand on a bench for support.
- With the other hand, lift a dumbbell from the floor to your side, keeping your back straight.
- Lower the dumbbell back to the starting position.
- Perform 3 sets of 10-12 repetitions per side.

Deadlifts

- Stand with feet hip-width apart, a barbell in front of your shins.
- Bend at the hips and knees to grip the bar with a shoulder-width grip.
- Keep your back flat, lift the bar by straightening your hips and knees.
- Lower the bar to the ground under control.
- Execute 3 sets of 6-8 repetitions.

3. Shoulders

Overhead Press

- Stand with feet shoulder-width apart, holding a barbell at shoulder level.
- Press the barbell overhead until arms are fully extended.
- Lower back to the start position.
- Do 3 sets of 8-10 repetitions.

Lateral Raises

- Stand with feet hip-width apart, dumbbells at your sides.
- With elbows slightly bent, raise the dumbbells to the side until they reach shoulder height.
- Lower them back down slowly.
- Complete 3 sets of 10-12 repetitions.

Front Raises

- Stand with feet hip-width apart, dumbbells in front of your thighs.
- Raise one dumbbell directly in front of you to shoulder height, keeping your arm straight.
- Lower it back down, and repeat with the other arm.
- Perform 3 sets of 10-12 repetitions per arm.

4. Legs

Squats

- Stand with feet a bit wider than shoulder-width apart.
- Bend your knees and hips to lower your body as if sitting in a chair.
- Keep your chest up and your back straight.
- Push through your heels to return to the starting position.
- Complete 3 sets of 10-12 repetitions.

Lunges

- Stand with feet together.
- Step forward with one leg and lower your body until both knees are bent at 90 degrees.
- Push back up to the starting position.
- Alternate legs, performing 3 sets of 10-12 repetitions per leg.

Leg Curls

- Lie face down on a leg curl machine with your ankles under the padded bar.
- Curl your legs up towards your buttocks as far as possible.
- Slowly return to the starting position.
- Perform 3 sets of 10-12 repetitions.

5. Core

Planks

- Lie face down on the floor.

- Raise yourself up onto your elbows and toes, keeping your body in a straight line from head to heels.

- Hold this position for 30 seconds to 1 minute.

- Perform 3 sets.

Russian Twists

- Sit on the floor with your knees bent and feet flat.

- Lean back slightly and lift your feet off the floor.

- Hold a medicine ball or weight and twist your torso from side to side.

- Do this motion for 30 seconds, rest, and repeat for 3 sets.

Bicycle Crunches

- Lie on your back with your hands behind your head and legs raised to form a 90-degree angle.

- Bring your right elbow to your left knee while straightening your right leg.

- Switch sides, bringing your left elbow to your right knee.

- Alternate sides in a pedaling motion for 20-30 repetitions for each set, aiming for 3 sets.

Tips for Low-Carb Day Workouts

- **Stay Hydrated**: Low-carb days might change how your body retains water, so ensure you drink plenty of water before, during, and after your workout.

- **Monitor Your Energy Levels**: Initially, you might feel less energetic on low-carb days. Adjust the intensity of workouts if necessary, but usually, energy levels adapt over time.

- **Warm-Up Properly**: Start with a good warm-up to reduce the risk of injuries. This is especially important as the body might take longer to warm up on a low-carb diet.

- **Focus on Form**: With potentially lowered energy, it's crucial to focus on maintaining proper form to maximize the effectiveness of each exercise and avoid injuries.

- **Cool Down and Stretch**: Conclude each session with a cool-down period and some stretching to aid in recovery and flexibility.

Exercises for High-Carb Days

The day after consuming a higher carbohydrate intake, blood glucose and muscle glycogen levels will be replenished. This fuels intense training and heavier lifting, which is not advisable on low carb days. On high carb days, select exercises that maximize power output and anabolic stimulus. Effective routines include:

- **Weight Training:** The restored glycogen enhances performance for heavier compound lifts like squats, deadlifts, and Olympic movements. Multiple sets of 3-5 reps build maximal strength and muscle mass. Use 2-5 minutes of rest between sets. Focus on large muscle groups and multi-joint lifts for optimal anabolic hormone response.

- **High Intensity Interval Training (HIIT):** Brief, repeated bouts of high intensity effort tap into glycolytic energy systems fueled by higher blood glucose levels. Sprints, rowing intervals, battling ropes, jump ropes, shuttle runs, or cycling sprints are great 30 second to 2 minute intervals. Push near maximal effort during the work intervals. Active rest 1-3 minutes between intervals. Limit HIIT sessions to 20-30 total minutes.

- **Power and Plyometrics Circuits:** Explosive medicine ball throws, box jumps, burpees, jump squats, and lateral bounds help develop power for sports. The full body drills follow circuits or timed intervals with short rest periods. Plyos both build and require power. Higher carbs provide the requisite fuel for these intense plyometric sessions.

- **Metabolic Resistance Training:** Hybrid lifts blending power, strength, and cardio burn glycogen stores while increasing conditioning. Perform complexes where you move quickly between exercises targeting upper, lower, and core muscles with minimal rest. Examples are thrusters into pull ups into lunges or lateral high pulls into push presses into burpees. Keep rest intervals under a minute between sets.

- **Barre and Cross Training:** High-energy formats like barre, cycling, dance, stepping, kickboxing, and rowing draw heavily on glycogen for cardio endurance and fast twitch muscle fibers. Higher carbs allow pushing through the burn during sustained effort. Incorporate a couple of these sustained, high-intensity classes weekly when glycogen is restored.

- **Climbs, Sprints, and Prowler Pushes:** Outdoor hill sprints, bleacher runs, and loaded sled/prowler pushes generate incredible metabolic burn and spike anabolic hormones post-training. Perform 3-8 all-out sprints up a steep grade. Full recovery between sprints ensures maximum power and effort. Higher muscle glycogen provides the energy to fuel these brutal bursts.

- **Team Sports or Games:** Higher carb intake provides fuel for competitive recreational sports like basketball, tennis, hockey, soccer, and ultimate frisbee. Partake in active games or practice drills on high-energy days to synergize nutrition and competitive performance. Have fun while torching extra carb calories.

Listen to your body's biofeedback on high days. If you feel low energy despite sufficient carbs, reduce volume, intensity, or duration accordingly. Proper intra-workout fuel like sports drinks provides carbs and electrolytes during lengthy training on high days. Emphasize protein and anti-inflammatory foods for recovery after.

Exercises for High-Carb Days PRACTICE

For High-Carb days, exercises should be oriented towards higher intensity and heavier muscle work, making use of the extra energy provided by carbohydrates.

1. Squats

Type: Strength

Instructions:

- Stand with feet slightly wider than shoulder-width apart.
- Lower down as if sitting in a chair until thighs are parallel to the floor.
- Keep your back straight and chest up.
- Push through your heels to return to the starting position.

Sets/Reps: 4 sets of 8-10 reps

2. Deadlifts

Type: Strength

Instructions:

- Stand with feet hip-width apart, barbell in front of you.
- Bend at your hips and knees, grab the bar with an overhand grip.
- Keep your back straight, lift the bar by straightening your hips and knees.
- Lower the bar back to the ground under control.

Sets/Reps: 3 sets of 6-8 reps

3. Bench Press

Type: Strength

Instructions:

- Lie back on a bench with a barbell positioned above your chest.
- Lower the bar slowly until it touches your mid-chest.
- Push the bar back up to the starting position.

Sets/Reps: 3 sets of 8 reps

4. Pull-Ups

Type: Strength/Endurance

Instructions:

- Hang from a pull-up bar with hands slightly wider than shoulder-width.
- Pull yourself up until your chin is over the bar.
- Lower yourself slowly back to the start.

Sets/Reps: As many as possible in 3 sets

5. Leg Press

Type: Strength

Instructions:

- Sit on a leg press machine with yourfeet shoulder-width apartt on the platform. sPress the platform away explosively, then return to the starting position under control.

Sets/Reps: 4 sets of 10 reps

6. Rowing Machine

Type: Cardio/Endurance

Instructions:

- Use a rowing machine at a challenging but sustainable pace.

- Focus on a smooth, continuous motion.

Duration: 20-30 minutes

Tips for High-Carb Day Workouts

- Fuel Properly: Since these are high-carb days, ensure you consume a good mix of carbs and protein before your workout to maximize energy levels.

- Stay Hydrated: High-intensity workouts on high-carb days can also mean more sweating. Keep hydrated to maintain performance.

- Focus on Form: With the heavier loads and higher intensity, maintaining proper form is crucial to avoid injuries.

Merry Lott

CHAPTER 4
MASTERING MEAL PREP AND KITCHEN ESSENTIALS

Essential Cooking Tools and Ingredients

Kitchen tools and ingredients simplify preparing delicious, nutritious meals that fit your carb cycling plan. Having the right basics on hand saves time while enabling you to whip up both keto and higher carb dishes easily. Invest in these essentials:

- **Quality set of pots and pans** - Stainless steel and ceramic coated pans evenly distribute heat without leaching chemicals. They also cook meat and vegetables without sticking. Have small and large saucepans, a skillet, and oven-safe options.

- **Set of sharp knives** - Sharp knives are safer and more efficient than dull ones for chopping, slicing, and dicing ingredients. An 8" chef's knife, paring knife,e and serrated bread knife cover most tasks. Invest in a sharpening stone or knife sharpener. Proper knife skills further expedite cooking.

- **Cutting boards** - Durable wooden or plastic cutting boards protect your knives and countertops. Have separate boards for produce and animal proteins to avoid cross-contamination. Bamboo boards have naturally antibacterial properties.

- **Mixing bowls** - Nesting glass or stainless steel bowls enables mixing, tossing salads,s and prep work. Microwave and freezer-safe options increase versatility. Measure ingredients right in mixing bowls.

- **Measuring cups and spoons** - Accurately portioning ingredients ensures recipes turn out right. Always level off dry ingredients with a knife for precision.

- **Food scale** - Weighing protein foods and dense ingredients like nut butter is more accurate than measuring cups. Scales help dial in macros and calories.

- **Whisk** - Hand held or electric whisks smoothly blend wet ingredients like eggs, batters, and dressings.

- **Spatulas and turners** - Flexible silicone spatulas enable cleanly scraping bowls and pans. Slotted turners flip proteins cleanly.

- **Tongs** - Grab and flip foods easily without piercing them. Protect pan coatings from damage.

- **Ladles and spoons** - Stainless spoons and ladles serve soups, stir pans, and handle both savory and sweet dishes.

- **Grater and zester** - Graters transform vegetables and hard cheeses into fluffy mounds for salads, baked dishes, andgarnishesh. Microplane zesters make flavorful citrus zest.

- **Vegetable peeler** - Quickly peel fruits and vegetables without waste.

- **Colander and strainer** - Rinse produce, drain boiled pasta/grains and separate liquid from solids.

- **Prep bowls** – Use separate prep bowls for chopped veggies, measured dry goods, and prepped proteins to stay organized.

- **Baking dishes and pans** - Metal and ceramic baking pans distribute oven heat evenly. Have multiple sizes.

- **Rimmed baking sheets** - Make oven roasting veggies and proteins easy. Line with parchment paper for quick cleanup.

- **Stand mixer** - Optional but invaluable for kneading dough and whipping creamed ingredients hands-free.

- **Immersion blender** - Purées soup and sauces right in pots and bowls for fast, smooth textures.

- **Slow cooker** - Dump ingredients in for effortless shredded meats, stews, and chili with little monitoring. Great for batch meals.

With handy tools and essential pantry items, you can cook carb cycling meals quickly and cleanly. Stock up on versatile fresh produce like onions, garlic, spinach, peppers, zucchini and mushrooms. Add eggs, meats, healthy fats, spices, broths, and condiments. Meal prepping saves more time while setting you up for carb cycling success.

Efficient Meal Prep Techniques

Achieving an optimal carb cycling routine requires dedicated meal preparation. Fortunately, proven strategies and techniques enable you to quickly batch cook protein, produce, and complex carbs for both low carb and high carb days. Here are some time-saving tips for efficient carb cycling meal prep:

- **Prep Proteins First** - Proteins take longest to cook. Oven roast season slabs of salmon, chicken breasts, or lean red meat on Sundays to use all week. Or fill your slow cooker with stew meat, chicken thighs or pork shoulder. Having precooked proteins on hand makes assembling meals fast.

- **Pre-Cook Vegetables** - Roast, sauté, or steam broccoli, cauliflower, zucchini, peppers and other vegetables in bulk too. Store them in containers to add to recipes or eat as snacks all week. They can go straight from fridge to plate.

- **Cook Once, Eat Twice** - Double recipes, then repurpose leftovers creatively. Shredded taco chicken transitions to a salad topping or soup. Roasted veggies become frittata fillings. Cooked lentils can make curry today, then stuff peppers tomorrow.

- **Stock Up On Staples** - Keep your pantry and fridge loaded with nuts, nut butter, olives, avocados, leafy greens, eggs, plant milks, frozen berries, and other versatile items. They quickly combine into meals.

- **Wash & Prep Produce** - Wash berries, chop veggies, and grate cheese during downtime to utilize them all week long without waste.

- **Make Large Batches** - Instead of one casserole or pot of soup, prepare two or three, then freeze individual portions for grab-and-go meals later.

- **Use Meal Delivery Kits** - To simplify, utilize pre-portioned meal kits on busy days. The ingredients come prepped and ready to cook with minimal effort.

- **Get Saucy** - Make extra marinara, pesto, and dressings to flavor up dishes all week. They add big taste fast.

- **Parcook Grains & Legumes** - Partially cook beans, quinoa, farro, and brown rice ahead in a large batch. Finish individual servings quickly as needed.

- **Embrace Batch Cooking** - Dedicate 2-3 hours on weekends to chop, cook, and assemble multiple dishes at once for the coming week. Playlist dance parties ease the chore.

- **Simplify With Sheet Pan Meals** - Pile veggies and protein on one sheet pan, then roast together. Minimal cleanup!

Planning ahead and utilizing time-saving batch cooking techniques lets you quickly assemble balanced carb cycling meals for an entire week. Just dedicate a couple of hours over the weekend to execute your meal prep plan. The investment pays off all week long.

Preserving Nutrients While Cooking

When preparing nutritious carb-cycling meals, retaining vitamins and minerals lost during cooking boosts the health impact. Luckily, research shows certain techniques maximize nutrient preservation in plant foods and animal proteins. Implement these evidence-based methods:

- **Steaming:** Unlike boiling, which leaches water-soluble vitamins, steaming gently cooks veggies and meats enveloped in moist heat. The indirect contact with boiling water preserves more B-complex vitamins like folate and biotin, along with vitamin C.

- **Microwaving:** Despite myths, zapping vegetables retains antioxidants and vitamins better than boiling due to shortened cook times. Microwaves only deplete certain heat-sensitive B-vitamins. However, high temperatures can still degrade other vitamins.

- **Baking and Roasting:** Dry cooking methods like baking and roasting avoid nutrient loss from immersion in water. Go low and slow to minimize damage to delicate vitamins. High temperatures will still degrade some nutrition. Cooking veggies with fats boosts the absorption of fat-soluble nutrients too.

- **Raw Plant Foods:** Eating produce like peppers, cucumbers, berries, leafy greens, and broccoli raw preserves all their delicate nutrients intact. But cooking increases the absorption of certain antioxidants like lycopene and carotenoids in tomatoes, carrots, and peppers. Light steaming is optimal for balancing raw enzymes with absorption.

- **Acidic Cooking:** Adding lemon, vinegar, tomatoes, or wine to cooking water counteracts alkalinity, which destroys water-soluble vitamins. Acidic environments preserve these during cooking.

- **Quick Cooking:** The longer the cooking time and exposure to heat, the greater the vitamin loss. Opt for fast sautéing, grilling, or roasting, and avoid prolonged boiling or baking.

- **Smaller Pieces:** Chopping veggies and meats into smaller pieces shortens the cooking duration, preserving more nutrients. Dicing or shredding carrots, zucchini, peppers, cabbage, etc. reduces cook times.

- **Low Liquid:** Boiling veggies in lots of water magnifies the leaching of water-soluble vitamins. Use minimal water for steaming or cooking grains and pasta. Restrict surface contact.

- **Dark Cooking Surfaces:** Using stainless steel, enameled, or ceramic cookware instead of aluminum, copper, or iron retains more nutrients during oven roasting or stovetop cooking.

- **Cooked Then Raw:** Enjoy cooked veggies like asparagus, green beans, or broccoli warm, then snack on raw leftovers to gain the benefits of both.

- **Leftovers:** Vitamin loss continues in cooked, refrigerated foods. Eat leftovers, like roasted veggies, within 3-4 days. Prioritize fresh-cooked foods.

- **Cooking Sprays:** Lightly coating pans with avocado, olive, or coconut oil spray prevents sticking while minimizing oxidation from high heat exposure.

- **Low Slow Cooking:** Extended braising, stewing, and slow cooking at low temperatures tenderizes meats while better retaining vitamin content.

- **Meat Juices:** Nutrients like iron and B-vitamins leach into cooking liquid. Utilize juices from cooked meat for gravies and sauces over dishes.

- **Vitamin Saving Herbs:** Rosemary, thyme, sage, and garlic contain compounds that combat vitamin loss during heating. Add these antioxidant herbs to recipes.

- **Soaking Beans:** Phytates in uncooked beans chelate and reduce minerals. Soaking then rinsing pinto, kidney, etc beans before cooking preserves more iron, calcium, and zinc while degrading fewer vitamins.

Adequate hydration also maximizes nutrient absorption. Drink water consistently while carb cycling. Follow these evidence-based techniques to preserve nutrition in home cooked fare.

Quick Fixes for Busy Days

Life gets hectic sometimes, making carb cycling prep challenging. With some clever hacks, you can still eat well on busy, time-crunched days. These quick fixes help maintain your regimen when you're overwhelmed and low on time:

- **Pre-chop Produce** - When you meal prep, chop extra veggies, fruits, and herbs to have ready for fast dishes later. Pre-cut peppers, onions, garlic, and greens enable throwing together meals in minutes.

- **Stock Your Freezer** - Cook and freeze batches of shredded chicken, lean beef crumbles, veggie burgers, soups, chilis, and casseroles on less busy weekends. Thaw and reheat for instant meals when frantic.

- **Leftovers Are Your Friend** - Double up on batch cooking. Repurpose leftovers for fast new meals later. Shredded taco meat, roasted veggies, and cooked grains reinvent easily.

- **Keep Snacks Handy** - Store nuts, seeds, nut butter packs, protein bars, jerky sticks, and portable fruits at home, at work, in your car, and in your gym bag. Healthy snacking saves time.

- **Leverage Rotisserie Chicken -** Grab pre-cooked rotisserie chickens from the grocery deli. Shred meat for salads, wraps, soups, or casseroles in minutes.

- **Mix and Match Veggies** - Frozen veggie mixes, pre-chopped fresh veggies, and salad bar selections make sides come together fast.

- **Quick-Cooking Grains** - Opt for fast-cooking grains like quinoa, amaranth, polenta, couscous, etc. Cook in just 10-15 minutes. Or make a big batch of rice on weekends for quick meals during the week.

- **Canned Beans** - No time to soak and simmer dried beans? Grab canned chickpeas, kidney, or black beans to instantly add protein, fiber, and nutrients to any dish.

- **Invest in a Slow Cooker** - Toss ingredients in the morning and come home to finished stews, chilis, and shredded meats for fast meal assembly at night.

- **Multitask in the Kitchen** - Take advantage of overlapping prep. Roast veggies while simmering grains. Cook proteins in batches while chopping produce for other meals.

- **Lean on Sheet Pan Meals** - Dump proteins and veggies on a sheet pan to roast together without much prep or cleanup. Easy one-pan cooking.

- **Prep On The Go** - Wash and chop produce during kids activities or while working from home. Bring Tupperware and knives to games and appointments.

- **Reinvent Leftovers** - Combine leftover proteins, grains, and veggies in creative new ways like burritos, rice bowls, stir fry, omelets, etc.

- **Prep Freeze Ahead** - Portion and freeze ingredients layered in foil packets for future dump and bake meals. Defrost and throw in the oven for fast homemade fare.

With the right strategies, you can eat well-balanced low-carb and high-carb meals even when life gets chaotic. A little advanced prep and planning goes a long way on hectic days.

CHAPTER 5
OVERCOMING CHALLENGES AND ADJUSTMENTS

Common Pitfalls and How to Overcome Them

Structuring your days around carb cycling takes planning and persistence. When life gets chaotic, you may run into common pitfalls. But knowledge of these stumbling blocks equips you to get quickly back on track:

- **Surprise social events** - Birthdays, happy hours, and date nights may spontaneously disrupt your carb schedule and meal prep. Accept that flexibility is key sometimes. Balance indulgence with recommitting to the plan the next day. Bring your own snacks or eat lightly beforehand.

- **Feeling deprived** - If you're fixated on the carbs you "can't" have, it fosters resentment and may lead to binges. Remind yourself that this is temporary. Focus on abundant anti-inflammatory whole foods you can enjoy.

- **Tracking burnout** - Weighing, measuring, and logging meals gets tedious. Take a few days off from tracking while still choosing compliant options. Or simplify by tracking just protein and total carbs.

- **Weekend splurges** - High-carb weekends derail fat loss plans. Schedule an active refeed day, but make smart swaps, watch portions, and limit alcohol. Get back on plan Sunday night.

- **Missing workouts** - When work, family, or illness interrupt training, be kind to yourself. Double up another day if possible, even with an active rest day when needed. Consistency over perfection.

- **Plateaus** - If progress stalls, ensure you're tracking accurately. Upping activity levels, changing exercise selection, and tweaking macros may refresh results. Patience pays off.

- **Temptation everywhere** - Birthdays, holidays, and happy hours test willpower constantly. Have a plan for parties: eat lightly beforehand, focus on protein first, and, limit liquid calories. Bring a dish you can eat.

- **Vacations and travel** - With prep and planning, you can maintain a carb cycling schedule on weekends away and on trips. Pack snacks, research local grocery stores, and scope out restaurant menus ahead online. Prioritize fun and spend extra time in the hotel gym. Balance indulgences with lighter choices. Return immediately to routine afterward. Even on vacations, make each meal an opportunity to nourish your body well.

- **Life happens** - Illness, injuries, work events, and family obligations interfere sometimes. Don't scrap the whole plan. Just get gently back on track as soon as you can, maybe with modifications like lighter weights or low-impact cardio. Listen to your body and be adaptable.

Progress isn't linear. Ups and downs are part of the journey. Cultivate self-compassion when you veer off course. Refocus with your end goal in mind. Consistency ultimately matters far more than perfection. You've got this!

Adapting the Diet to Your Lifestyle

The beauty of carb cycling is its flexibility to adapt to diverse lifestyles and needs. Whether you're an athlete, office worker, stay-at-home parent, or frequent traveler, optimizing the diet around your routine improves sustainability and results. Consider your unique context:

Athletes & Active People

The demands of training and competition alter carb needs. Time high carb days around labor-intensive workouts for maximizing glycogen stores. Save fat-burning low-carb days for rest days or lighter training. Add carbs around competitions for optimal performance. Consume carb-focused meals or shakes immediately post-workout when your body rapidly absorbs carbs to replenish glycogen. Getting sufficient overall calories ensures you build lean mass.

Office Workers

If exercise happens after work, a small, high-carb afternoon snack fires up energy levels for hitting the gym after sedentary office hours. Pack carb-cycling-friendly lunches and snacks to resist vending machine temptation. Get steps in with short walk breaks. Standing or treadmill desks boost calorie burn at work. Schedule evening workouts, and you'll look forward to a delicious high-carb dinner as a reward.

Stay-at-Home Parents

Nurturing little ones all day is physically and mentally draining, making healthy habits tough. Prep filling, diet-compliant snacks like veggies and hummus, cottage cheese, nuts, or apples with nut butter for grab-and-go energy to keep you fueled on busy parenting days. Do as much activity with the kids as you can - go on walks, bike rides, and hikes. Use their nap time for a re-energizing workout. Enjoy carb-rich meals together as a family.

Frequent Travelers

With planning, carb cycling works anywhere. Scope out grocery stores at your destination to buy produce, proteins, and healthy fats for DIY meals. Pack non-perishable snacks like nuts, protein bars, and pouches of olives, nut butters, or tuna. Research nearby gyms or studios to maintain workout routines. Choose hotel rooms with kitchenettes for preparing meals. At restaurants, modify dishes by replacing carbs with extra vegetables.

Shift Workers

Erratic schedules disrupt circadian rhythms, affecting weight control and performance. Stick with wholesome, balanced meals as much as possible. Keep portable snacks on hand for odd hours when you can't prep food. Get exercise when you can, especially on mornings or nights off to maintain fitness. Nap during the day if working overnight. Stay hydrated and listen to your body's needs.

Getting Started

If diving into full blown carb cycling seems intimidating, ease into it. Gradually reduce overall carb portions for a week or two, then shift higher carb meals to workout days. Build up from lighter 20-30 minute workouts to longer HIIT sessions as fitness improves. Modify the diet flexibly until you find a comfortable groove. Give your body time to adapt.

No matter your demands, tailoring carb cycling strategies to your individual lifestyle leads to sustainable success and optimal wellbeing. Remain patient, adaptable, and compassionate with yourself. This journey is all about progress over perfection.

How to Handle Social Situations and Dining Out

Social events and restaurants often derail healthy habits, but with preparation, carb cycling can adapt. Follow these proven tips for navigating gatherings and eating out while staying on track:

Attending Parties

Holiday gatherings, birthday bashes, and cocktail fêtes are ubiquitous. With planning, though, they don't have to sabotage your efforts.

- Before arriving, consume a balanced meal emphasizing protein, healthy fats, and vegetables. Going in satiated, curbs cravings and overindulging. Bring an appetizer you can eat, like vegetable crudités.

- Survey the buffet first before filling your plate. Focus on lean proteins, fresh fruits and veggies, and small servings of whole grains. Limit starchy sides, sugary desserts, and liquid calories from alcohol or soda.

- If noshing all evening, go for vegetable-based options first, then modest portions of proteins and smart carbs like quinoa salad or lentil dishes. Fill up half your plate with salad.

- Politely decline pushy hosts urging you to try heavy foods. Have a strategy for indulgence, like one small taste. Savor it mindfully, then get back on track. Or politely explain your dietary needs.

- Enjoy conversation and company first, not constant grazing. Step away from temptation periodically for some fresh air or mingling instead of lingering by the buffet.

- Bring along a tasty herbal tea or infused water as an alternative to alcohol or sugary drinks. Staying hydrated prevents overdoing it on food.

Eating at Restaurants

Dining out requires additional diligence to stay carb-cycling compliant. With some modifications, you can succeed anywhere from fast casual to fine dining establishments.

- Peruse menus in advance online and decide what you'll order before arriving hungry and tempted. Seek out mains with lean proteins, veggies, and healthy fats.

- Ask how dishes are prepared. Request extra modifications, like getting sauces and dressings on the side. Most restaurants happily oblige customers' requests.

- Prioritize grilled, baked, broiled, or poached cooking methods instead of fried. Seek creative substitutions, like cauliflower rice, instead of starchy sides.

- Don't feel obligated to finish oversized portions, which are typical at most eateries nowadays. Take a portion home for tomorrow's lunch.

- Balance indulgences like that basket of warm bread or artisanal pasta dish with making the rest of the meal veggie-centric.

- For beverages, stick with unsweetened iced tea, a splash of wine, or mineral water with lemon instead of sugary cocktails or calorie-laden lattes.

- Feel empowered, not embarrassed, by asking questions and making special requests. Don't apologize for personalized needs. Servers won't mind modifying dishes.

- If dining with a group, others may order indulgent fare. Don't let it influence your choices for your own health goals. Order thoughtfully.

- On vacation, away from your routine, enjoy local flavors in moderation without totally abandoning the structure that has gotten you results. Get back on track after.

Social and restaurant situations require forethought and flexibility for smart choices. But with the right mindset and strategies, you can still make progress, one delicious meal at a time.

Adjusting the Carb Cycling Plan for Continuous Improvement

Carb cycling only produces desirable long-term results if implemented as an adaptable lifestyle, not a rigid short-term diet. As your body and needs change, alter the plan to optimize it. Consistently monitor energy, hunger, cravings, body composition, and workout performance. Then tweak variables to feel your best and see ongoing progress.

Fine-tuning macros:

Play with your carb and fat ratios based on how you feel overall and your body's response. If you feel lethargic and are losing strength on workout days, add more carbs. Increase fat if you feel constantly hungry between meals. Adjust macros in 5-10 gram increments each week to find your personal sweet spot.

Modifying high days vs low days:

If you aren't seeing desired fat loss results, add an extra low-carb day, swapping out a high-carb day. Or increase the carb differential between high and low days for greater caloric fluctuation. If you're irritable, stressed, and lacking energy for workouts, add a high-carb day back in or increase high-day carbs.

Changing training:

Plateaus happen, especially if you follow an exercise routine for many weeks on end. Shift your workout style, intensity, frequency, or duration to re-ignite results. Take a break from heavy lifting to focus on athletic training like sprints, circuits, or conditioning for a couple weeks. Or enjoy new active hobbies like rock climbing, hiking, or recreation league sports.

Recalculating calories:

If the scale won't budge, recheck your total daily calories and adjust up or down by 200-400 as needed for continual weight loss, maintenance, or gain goals. Our metabolic needs change over time.

Improving nutrition quality:

The longer you eat well, the more your tastebuds adapt to appreciate whole foods. Gradually keep increasing produce, decreasing packaged snacks, and focusing on simple preparations to crowd out cravings. Cleaner eating means better wellness and body composition.

Paying attention to timing:

Sync your carb intake with your unique schedule and body rhythms for optimal energy and sleep. If after dinner carbs disrupt your sleep, eat them earlier. If you're exhausted midday, add more carbs at lunch. Timing your meals and macros intelligently prevents crashes, cravings, and burnout.

Knowing when to take a break:

Rigidity is not sustainable long-term. If you're feeling overly stressed, restricted, or burnt out from diligent carb cycling, take a week at maintenance calories with balanced macronutrients and intuitive eating. Recalibrate with rest and recovery. Come back feeling recharged and refocused.

Celebrating milestones:

Use each goal met as an opportunity to enjoy your favorite treats in moderation. Savor some pizza or ice cream after hitting a bodyweight or strength PR. Then get immediately back on track. Reward yourself for wins along the journey.

Carb cycling must mold to your needs as they change over time. Regularly assess energy, body composition, and workouts to make small but impactful adjustments that keep you progressing. Consistency with flexibility is key. This is a personalized marathon, not a sprint.

Motivational Tips to Keep You Going

Any lifestyle change presents challenges that can derail progress if you lose motivation. But lasting transformation relies on perseverance and perspective shifts. Use these strategies to stay inspired, empowered, and on track:

Visualize the end goal

When tempted to stray, get clear on your motivations. Revisit pictures of your dream body or envision finally reaching fitness milestones. Keep your eye on the prize - this short-term sacrifice leads to huge payoffs if you stick it out. Let your big-picture purpose renew your commitment.

Progress over perfection

Don't beat yourself up over small slip-ups. Minor indulgences and missed workouts are inevitable. Expect setbacks, and be resilient. Every choice is a chance to get right back on track. String together consistent days, not perfect days, for results.

Focus on how you'll feel

Dwell not on what you can't eat, but on all the wholesome, nourishing foods that make you feel energized and vibrant. Shift from a restriction mentality to thoughts of gaining health, strength, and confidence.

Celebrate small wins

Note even tiny victories like passing on office donuts, choosing salad over fries, waking up for an early workout. Reward yourself with non-food treats for sticking to the plan. Track milestones to reinforce achievements.

Find your motivation style

We each need different types of motivation. Some rely on inspiration from others' success stories. Some need gentle accountability from a coach or buddy. Others find motivation internally through self-discipline and belief in themselves. Know your motivational style and nurture it.

Pass on "all or nothing" thoughts

Trying to be perfect with zero slip-ups backfires. Eliminate unhelpful black and white thinking. After a bad meal, don't throw in the towel, thinking you already ruined your diet. Just resume with the very next meal. Progress comes from keeping going.

Make it fun

Inject enjoyment into your program so it never feels like drudgery. Discover new recipes to prevent taste fatigue. Get creative with meal prep presentations. Make exercise social and bond with loved ones over active hobbies. Gamify your routine and track your wins.

Focus on adding, not depriving

This isn't about restriction but about experiencing all the glorious whole foods that make you thrive. Add in more fresh produce, fun ways to move, quality time with others, and immersing yourself in hobbies. A full, vibrant life is the ultimate motivation.

Look beyond the scale

While the numbers may fluctuate, the big payoff is what this achieves: health, confidence, strength, discipline, and self-respect. Appreciate all the non-scale victories. They reveal your true progress.

Enjoy the journey

Don't just fixate on the destination, savor the process. Find happiness in preparing wholesome meals, connecting mind and body through movement, and building lifelong healthy habits. Let the path enrich you as much as crossing the finish line.

Stay open and solution-focused when obstacles arise. Maintain hope that progress comes little by little. With patience and care for yourself, the small steps add up to big transformations. You've got what it takes to succeed. Enjoy the ride!

CHAPTER 6
LOW-CARB RECIPES

Low-Carb Breakfasts

1. Avocado and Egg Toast

Preparation Time: 10 minutes

Cooking Time: 5 minutes

Ingredients:

1 large avocado

2 eggs

2 slices of low-carb bread

Salt and pepper to taste

Chopped parsley (for garnish)

Preparation:

- Toast the low-carb bread slices.
- While the bread is toasting, fry or poach the eggs to your liking.
- Mash the avocado and spread evenly on each slice of toast.
- Top each with an egg, season with salt, pepper, and garnish with parsley.

Benefits:

It provides a balance of healthy fats, protein, and fiber; great for energy and satiety.

2. Greek Yogurt and Nut Parfait

Preparation Time: 5 minutes

Cooking Time: 0 minutes

Ingredients:

1 cup full-fat Greek yogurt

1/4 cup mixed nuts (almonds, walnuts, pecans), roughly chopped

1 tbsp chia seeds

1 tsp vanilla extract

Preparation:

- In a bowl, mix the Greek yogurt with vanilla extract.
- In serving glasses, layer half the yogurt, then a layer of mixed nuts and chia seeds.
- Repeat the layers, and serve.

Benefits:

High in protein and healthy fats, aiding in muscle repair and providing a long-lasting energy source.

3. Spinach and Feta Omelette

Preparation Time: 5 minutes

Cooking Time: 10 minutes

Ingredients:

4 eggs

1 cup fresh spinach

1/2 cup feta cheese, crumbled

1 tbsp olive oil

Salt and pepper to taste

Preparation:

- Beat the eggs in a bowl and season with salt and pepper.
- Heat olive oil in a skillet over medium heat; sauté spinach until wilted.
- Pour the eggs over the spinach and sprinkle feta cheese on top.
- Cook until the eggs are set, and fold the omelette before serving.

Benefits:

Rich in protein and calcium, and the spinach provides iron and vitamins for a strong start to the day.

4. Smoked Salmon and Cream Cheese Roll-Ups

Preparation Time: 10 minutes

Cooking Time: 0 minutes

Ingredients:

4 oz smoked salmon

2 oz cream cheese, softened

1 tbsp capers

1 tbsp dill, chopped

4 large lettuce leaves

Preparation:

- Spread cream cheese on each lettuce leaf.
- Top with smoked salmon, sprinkle with capers and dill.
- Roll up the lettuce leaves tightly and slice into bite-sized pieces.

Benefits:

It offers a good source of omega-3 fatty acids and protein, promoting heart health and muscle growth.

5. Chia Seed Pudding

Preparation Time: 5 minutes (+ soaking overnight)

Cooking Time: 0 minutes

Ingredients:

1/4 cup chia seeds

1 cup unsweetened almond milk

1/2 tsp vanilla extract

1 tbsp almond butter

1 tbsp sugar-free maple syrup (optional)

Preparation:

- In a bowl, mix together chia seeds, almond milk, and vanilla extract.
- Let it sit overnight in the refrigerator to thicken.
- Stir in almond butter and maple syrup before serving.

Benefits:

High in fiber and omega-3 fatty acids, which are great for digestion and cardiovascular health.

6. Cauliflower Hash Browns

Preparation Time: 10 minutes

Cooking Time: 15 minutes

Ingredients:

2 cups cauliflower, grated

1 egg

1/4 cup shredded cheddar cheese

1/4 cup finely chopped onion

Salt and pepper to taste

2 tbsp olive oil

Preparation:

- Combine grated cauliflower, egg, cheese, onion, salt, and pepper in a bowl.
- Heat olive oil in a skillet over medium heat.
- Scoop mixture into the skillet, flatten into a hash brown shape, and cook until golden brown on both sides.

Benefits:

Low in carbs, high in fiber, and provides a great alternative to traditional potato hash browns, supporting weight management.

7. Almond Flour Pancakes

Preparation Time: 10 minutes

Cooking Time: 15 minutes

Ingredients:

1 cup almond flour

2 eggs

1/3 cup water

1 tbsp olive oil

1 tsp baking powder

2 tbsp erythritol (or another sugar substitute)

1/2 tsp vanilla extract

Preparation:

- Whisk together all ingredients until smooth.
- Heat a non-stick skillet over medium heat and pour batter to form small pancakes.
- Cook until bubbles form on the surface, then flip and cook the other side.

Benefits:

Gluten-free and low in carbs, rich in protein and healthy fats, ideal for maintaining energy levels throughout the morning.

8. Coconut Flour Porridge

Preparation Time: 2 minutes

Cooking Time: 5 minutes

Ingredients:

2 tbsp coconut flour

1 cup coconut milk

1 tbsp flaxseed meal

Pinch of salt

Optional toppings: cinnamon, nuts, or berries

Preparation:

- In a small pot, combine coconut flour, flaxseed meal, salt, and coconut milk.
- Cook over medium heat while stirring continuously until it thickens.
- Serve with your choice of toppings.

Benefits:

High in fiber and healthy fats, supports digestive health and provides a slow release of energy.

9. Zucchini and Bell Pepper Frittata

Preparation Time: 10 minutes

Cooking Time: 20 minutes

Ingredients:

4 eggs

1 zucchini, sliced

1 bell pepper, diced

1/4 cup grated Parmesan cheese

1 tbsp olive oil

Salt and pepper to taste

Preparation:

- Preheat the oven to 375°F (190°C).
- Beat the eggs and mix with salt, pepper, and Parmesan.
- Sauté zucchini and bell pepper in olive oil over medium heat until soft.
- Pour the egg mixture over the vegetables and cook for a few minutes without stirring.
- Transfer the skillet to the oven and bake until the frittata is set.

Benefits:

It provides a good mix of vegetables and protein, enhancing muscle repair and overall health.

10. Bacon and Mushroom Scrambled Eggs

Preparation Time: 5 minutes

Cooking Time: 10 minutes

Ingredients:

4 eggs

4 slices of bacon, chopped

1/2 cup mushrooms, sliced

1 tbsp butter

Salt and pepper to taste

Preparation:

- In a skillet, cook bacon over medium heat until crispy.
- Add mushrooms and cook until soft.
- Beat eggs, salt, and pepper together and pour into the skillet with bacon and mushrooms.
- Stir gently until the eggs are fully cooked.

Benefits:

A satisfying meal providing high-quality protein and essential nutrients, perfect for a low-carb diet.

Low-Carb Lunches

1. Chicken Caesar Salad

Preparation Time: 15 minutes

Cooking Time: 10 minutes

Ingredients:

2 chicken breasts, grilled and sliced

4 cups Romaine lettuce, chopped

1/4 cup Parmesan cheese, shaved

2 tablespoons Caesar dressing, sugar-free

1 teaspoon olive oil

Salt and pepper to taste

Preparation:

- Season chicken breasts with salt and pepper, grill until fully cooked, and slice.
- Toss Romaine lettuce with Caesar dressing, top with chicken slices and Parmesan cheese.

Benefits:

High in protein, promotes muscle maintenance and satiety.

2. Zucchini Noodle Stir-Fry

Preparation Time: 10 minutes

Cooking Time: 10 minutes

Ingredients:

2 medium zucchinis, spiralized

1 bell pepper, sliced

1/2 onion, sliced

1 carrot, julienned

2 tablespoons soy sauce (low sodium)

1 tablespoon sesame oil

1 garlic clove, minced

1 teaspoon ginger, grated

Preparation:

- Heat sesame oil in a pan over medium heat. Add garlic and ginger, sauté for 1 minute.

- Add onion, bell pepper, and carrot, stir-fry for about 5 minutes.
- Add zucchini noodles and soy sauce, stir-fry for another 3-4 minutes until vegetables are tender but crisp.

Benefits:

Rich in vitamins and minerals, low in carbs, and perfect for energy stability.

3. Grilled Salmon with Asparagus

Preparation Time: 5 minutes

Cooking Time: 15 minutes

Ingredients:

2 salmon fillets

1 bunch asparagus, ends trimmed

2 tablespoons olive oil

Lemon wedges for serving

Salt and pepper to taste

Preparation:

- Preheat grill to medium-high.
- Brush salmon and asparagus with olive oil, season with salt and pepper.
- Grill salmon and asparagus for about 6-7 minutes per side, until salmon is flaky and asparagus is tender.
- Serve with lemon wedges.

Benefits:

Omega-3 fatty acids in salmon support heart health and cognitive function.

4. Cobb Salad

Preparation Time: 15 minutes

Cooking Time: 0 minutes

Ingredients:

4 cups mixed greens (lettuce, spinach, arugula)

1/2 cup cooked bacon, crumbled

2 hard-boiled eggs, sliced

1 avocado, diced

1/2 cup cherry tomatoes, halved

1/4 cup blue cheese, crumbled

2 tablespoons ranch dressing, sugar-free

Preparation:

- Arrange mixed greens in a large bowl.

- Top with rows of bacon, eggs, avocado, tomatoes, and blue cheese.
- Drizzle with ranch dressing before serving.

Benefits:

High in protein and healthy fats, helps fuel your body and keeps you full.

5. Beef and Broccoli

Preparation Time: 10 minutes

Cooking Time: 15 minutes

Ingredients:

300g beef strips

2 cups broccoli florets

1 tablespoon olive oil

2 cloves garlic, minced

1/4 cup beef broth

2 tablespoons soy sauce (low sodium)

1 teaspoon sesame oil

Preparation:

- In a large pan, heat olive oil over medium heat and sauté garlic until fragrant.
- Add beef strips and cook until browned.
- Add broccoli, beef broth, and soy sauce. Cover and simmer until broccoli is tender.
- Drizzle with sesame oil before serving.

Benefits:

Rich in protein and iron, essential for muscle repair and energy levels.

6. Turkey Lettuce Wraps

Preparation Time: 10 minutes

Cooking Time: 10 minutes

Ingredients:

300g ground turkey

1 bell pepper, diced

1/2 onion, diced

6 large lettuce leaves (such as iceberg or romaine)

1 tablespoon olive oil

2 tablespoons hoisin sauce, sugar-free

Salt and pepper to taste

Preparation:

- Heat olive oil in a skillet over medium heat. Add onion and bell pepper, sauté until soft.
- Add ground turkey, season with salt and pepper, and cook until browned.
- Stir in hoisin sauce and cook for another 2 minutes.
- Spoon the turkey mixture into lettuce leaves and serve.

Benefits:

Low in carbs and calories, high in protein, ideal for weight loss and maintaining lean muscle mass.

7. Avocado and Egg Salad

Preparation Time: 10 minutes

Cooking Time: 0 minutes

Ingredients:

2 hard-boiled eggs, chopped

1 ripe avocado, diced

1 tablespoon mayonnaise, sugar-free

1 teaspoon mustard

Salt and pepper to taste

2 tablespoons chopped chives

Preparation:

- In a bowl, combine eggs, avocado, mayonnaise, and mustard.
- Season with salt and pepper and mix gently.
- Sprinkle with chives before serving.

Benefits:

Rich in healthy fats and protein, supports cardiovascular health and fullness.

8. Shrimp and Avocado Salad

Preparation Time: 10 minutes

Cooking Time: 5 minutes

Ingredients:

200g shrimp, peeled and deveined

1 large avocado, sliced

1/2 cucumber, sliced

1/4 red onion, thinly sliced

2 tablespoons olive oil

Juice of 1 lime

Salt and pepper to taste

Preparation:

- Heat 1 tablespoon of olive oil over medium heat and cook shrimp until pink and opaque.
- In a salad bowl, combine cooked shrimp, avocado, cucumber, and red onion.
- Drizzle with remaining olive oil and lime juice. Season with salt and pepper.
- Toss gently and serve.

Benefits:

Packed with omega-3 fatty acids and antioxidants, promotes heart health and reduces inflammation.

9. Spinach and Feta Stuffed Chicken

Preparation Time: 15 minutes

Cooking Time: 25 minutes

Ingredients:

2 chicken breasts

1 cup fresh spinach, chopped

1/2 cup feta cheese, crumbled

1 garlic clove, minced

2 tablespoons olive oil

Salt and pepper to taste

Preparation:

- Preheat oven to 375°F (190°C).
- Make a pocket in each chicken breast and stuff with spinach, feta, and minced garlic.
- Season with salt and pepper, and seal with toothpicks.
- Heat olive oil in a skillet over medium heat and sear chicken on both sides until golden.
- Transfer to the oven and bake for 20 minutes, or until cooked through.

Benefits:

High in protein and calcium, supports bone health and muscle function.

10. Cauliflower Fried Rice

Preparation Time: 10 minutes

Cooking Time: 10 minutes

Ingredients:

1 head cauliflower, grated into 'rice'

1/2 cup mixed vegetables (peas, carrots, corn)

1/2 onion, diced

2 eggs, beaten

2 tablespoons soy sauce (low sodium)

1 tablespoon sesame oil

Salt and pepper to taste

Preparation:

- Heat sesame oil in a large skillet or wok over medium heat.
- Add onion and sauté until translucent.
- Add mixed vegetables and cook for 3 minutes.
- Stir in cauliflower rice and soy sauce, cook for 5 minutes.
- Push rice to the side, pour beaten eggs into the skillet, and scramble.
- Mix everything together, and season with salt and pepper.

Benefits:

Low in calories and carbs, high in fiber, aids in digestion and weight management.

11. Lemon Herb Grilled Chicken

Preparation Time: 15 minutes + marinating

Cooking Time: 20 minutes

Ingredients:

2 chicken breasts

2 tablespoons olive oil

Juice of 1 lemon

1 teaspoon dried herbs (thyme, oregano)

1 garlic clove, minced

Salt and pepper to taste

Preparation:

- In a bowl, mix olive oil, lemon juice, dried herbs, garlic, salt, and pepper.
- Marinate the chicken in the mixture for at least 30 minutes.
- Preheat grill to medium-high and grill chicken for about 10 minutes per side until fully cooked.

Benefits:

Low in fat and high in protein, it supports muscle growth and immune health with a boost from vitamin C in lemon.

12. Tuna Salad Stuffed Avocados

Preparation Time: 10 minutes

Cooking Time: 0 minutes

Ingredients:

1 can tuna, drained

2 avocados, halved and pitted

1/4 cup mayonnaise, sugar-free

1 celery stalk, finely chopped

1 tablespoon lemon juice

Salt and pepper to taste

Preparation:

- In a bowl, mix tuna, mayonnaise, celery, lemon juice, salt, and pepper.
- Scoop out some of the avocado from the halves to create space.
- Fill avocado halves with tuna mixture.

Benefits:

Rich in omega-3 fatty acids and healthy fats, promotes cardiovascular health and brain function.

13. Bacon and Spinach-stuffed Stuffed Mushrooms

Preparation Time: 15 minutes

Cooking Time: 20 minutes

Ingredients:

6 large portobello mushrooms, stems removed

1/2 cup cooked bacon, crumbled

1 cup spinach, sautéed and drained

1/2 cup cream cheese, softened

1/4 cup grated Parmesan cheese

Salt and pepper to taste

Preparation:

- Preheat oven to 350°F (175°C).
- In a bowl, mix bacon, spinach, cream cheese, Parmesan, salt, and pepper.
- Stuff mushroom caps with the mixture and place on a baking sheet.
- Bake for 20 minutes or until mushrooms are tender.

Benefits:

Provides a good source of protein, calcium, and antioxidants.

14. Greek Chicken Bowls

Preparation Time: 20 minutes

Cooking Time: 15 minutes

Ingredients:

2 chicken breasts, cubed

1 cucumber, diced

1/2 cup cherry tomatoes, halved

1/4 cup feta cheese, crumbled

1/4 cup olives, sliced

1 tablespoon olive oil

1 teaspoon Greek seasoning

Juice of 1 lemon

Preparation:

- Heat olive oil in a pan over medium heat and cook chicken with Greek seasoning until golden and cooked through.
- In a bowl, combine cucumber, cherry tomatoes, olives, and lemon juice.
- Serve chicken over the salad mixture and top with feta cheese.

Benefits:

High in protein and healthy fats, supports weight management and cardiovascular health.

15. Spicy Shrimp and Cauliflower Grits

Preparation Time: 10 minutes

Cooking Time: 15 minutes

Ingredients:

200g shrimp, peeled and deveined

1 head cauliflower, grated into 'grits'

1 cup chicken broth

1/2 cup cream cheese

1 tablespoon Cajun seasoning

1 garlic clove, minced

1 tablespoon olive oil

Preparation:

- In a pan, heat olive oil over medium heat, add garlic, and sauté for 1 minute.
- Add shrimp and Cajun seasoning, cook until shrimp are pink and cooked through.

- In another pan, simmer cauliflower grits in chicken broth until tender.
- Stir in cream cheese until smooth and creamy.
- Serve shrimp over cauliflower grits.

Benefits:

Low-carb alternative to traditional grits, high in protein and essential vitamins.

16. Beef Lettuce Wraps

Preparation Time: 15 minutes

Cooking Time: 10 minutes

Ingredients:

1 lb ground beef, lean

1 tablespoon soy sauce

1 garlic clove, minced

1 teaspoon ginger, grated

1 head of lettuce, leaves separated

1 carrot, julienned

1/2 cucumber, julienned

1/4 cup chopped green onions

1 tablespoon sesame oil

Preparation:

- Heat sesame oil in a pan over medium heat. Add garlic and ginger, sauté for 1 minute.
- Add ground beef, breaking it apart with a spatula. Cook until browned.
- Stir in soy sauce and cook for another 2 minutes.
- Lay lettuce leaves on a plate, spoon the cooked beef onto each leaf, top with carrot, cucumber, and green onions.
- Wrap the lettuce around the filling and serve.

Benefits:

This dish is low in carbs and high in protein, promoting muscle maintenance and growth. The fresh vegetables provide essential vitamins and minerals, supporting overall health.

17. Zucchini Noodles with Pesto

Preparation Time: 10 minutes

Cooking Time: 5 minutes

Ingredients:

4 medium zucchinis, spiralized

1/2 cup homemade or store-bought pesto

1/4 cup pine nuts, toasted

1/2 cup cherry tomatoes, halved

Salt and pepper to taste

Preparation:

- In a large pan, heat the pesto over medium heat.
- Add the spiralized zucchini and toss to coat with the pesto for about 2-3 minutes, just until the noodles are slightly softened.
- Remove from heat, add cherry tomatoes, and toss again.
- Season with salt and pepper, sprinkle with toasted pine nuts, and serve immediately.

Benefits:

Low in carbohydrates and calories. Zucchini provides dietary fiber, which aids in digestion. Pesto adds healthy fats and vitamins from basil and olive oil.

18. Coconut Curry Shrimp

Preparation Time: 10 minutes

Cooking Time: 15 minutes

Ingredients:

1 lb shrimp, peeled and deveined

1 tablespoon coconut oil

1 onion, finely chopped

2 garlic cloves, minced

1 tablespoon ginger, grated

1 can (14 oz) coconut milk

2 tablespoons curry powder

1 teaspoon turmeric

1/2 teaspoon cayenne pepper (adjust to taste)

Salt to taste

Fresh cilantro, chopped for garnish

Juice of 1 lime

Preparation:

- Heat coconut oil in a large skillet over medium heat. Add onion, garlic, and ginger, sautéing until onion is translucent.
- Stir in curry powder, turmeric, and cayenne pepper, cooking for about 1 minute until fragrant.
- Pour in the coconut milk, bringing the mixture to a simmer.

- Add the shrimp to the skillet, cooking until they are pink and fully cooked, about 5-7 minutes.
- Season with salt, and finish with lime juice.
- Garnish with fresh cilantro before serving.

Benefits:

This dish is rich in protein and healthy fats from the coconut milk, which can help improve heart health and boost the immune system. The spices used are great for inflammation and overall health.

Low-Carb Dinners

1. Zesty Lemon Garlic Salmon

Preparation Time: 10 minutes

Cooking Time: 20 minutes

Ingredients:

2 salmon fillets (6 oz each)

2 tablespoons olive oil

2 cloves garlic, minced

Juice and zest of 1 lemon

Salt and pepper to taste

1 tablespoon chopped fresh dill

Preparation:

- Preheat oven to 400°F (200°C).
- In a small bowl, mix olive oil, garlic, lemon juice, lemon zest, salt, and pepper.
- Place the salmon on a baking sheet lined with parchment paper. Pour the lemon garlic mixture over the salmon.
- Bake for 20 minutes or until the salmon flakes easily with a fork.
- Garnish with fresh dill before serving.

Benefits:

Rich in omega-3 fatty acids and lean protein, this dish supports heart health and muscle maintenance. The low-carb profile aids in fat loss phases.

2. Cauliflower Steak with Herb Pesto

Preparation Time: 15 minutes

Cooking Time: 25 minutes

Ingredients:

1 large head cauliflower

2 tablespoons olive oil

Salt and pepper to taste

For the pesto:

1 cup fresh basil leaves

1/4 cup pine nuts

2 cloves garlic

1/4 cup grated Parmesan cheese

1/2 cup olive oil

Salt to taste

Preparation:

- Preheat oven to 425°F (220°C).
- Slice cauliflower into 1/2 inch thick steaks. Brush both sides with olive oil, and season with salt and pepper.
- Place on a baking sheet and roast for about 25 minutes, flipping halfway through, until golden and tender.
- For the pesto, blend basil, pine nuts, garlic, Parmesan, and olive oil in a food processor until smooth. Season with salt.
- Serve cauliflower steaks topped with herb pesto.

Benefits:

Low in carbs and high in dietary fiber, this meal enhances digestive health, while the healthy fats in the pesto support cognitive function.

3. Spicy Chicken Lettuce Wraps

Preparation Time: 20 minutes

Cooking Time: 10 minutes

Ingredients:

1 lb chicken breast, minced

1 tablespoon olive oil

2 cloves garlic, minced

1 red bell pepper, diced

1 jalapeño, seeded and finely chopped

1 teaspoon chili powder

1/2 teaspoon cumin

Salt to taste

8-10 large lettuce leaves

Fresh cilantro for garnish

Preparation:

- Heat olive oil in a skillet over medium heat. Add garlic, bell pepper, and jalapeño, sautéing until soft.
- Add minced chicken, chili powder, cumin, and salt. Cook until chicken is browned and cooked through.
- Spoon the chicken mixture into lettuce leaves and garnish with fresh cilantro.

Benefits:

This dish is high in protein and low in carbs, making it ideal for muscle repair and fat loss. The spicy ingredients can boost metabolism.

4. Grilled Portobello Mushrooms with Almond Crust

Preparation Time: 10 minutes

Cooking Time: 15 minutes

Ingredients:

4 large Portobello mushroom caps

2 tablespoons olive oil

Salt and pepper to taste

1/2 cup almonds, finely chopped

2 tablespoons grated Parmesan cheese

1 clove garlic, minced

Preparation:

- Preheat grill to medium-high heat.
- Brush both sides of the mushroom caps with olive oil and season with salt and pepper.
- In a bowl, combine chopped almonds, Parmesan cheese, and minced garlic.
- Press the almond mixture onto the top side of each mushroom.
- Grill mushrooms, crust side up, for about 7-8 minutes, then carefully flip and grill for another 7 minutes or until tender.

Benefits:

High in healthy fats and low in carbs, this dish supports heart health and weight management. Mushrooms offer a meat-like texture, making this a satisfying meal for vegetarians.

5. Lemon Herb Grilled Shrimp

Preparation Time: 10 minutes (plus 30 minutes for marinating)

Cooking Time: 6 minutes

Ingredients:

1 lb shrimp, peeled and deveined

3 tablespoons olive oil

Juice and zest of 1 lemon

1 tablespoon chopped fresh parsley

1 clove garlic, minced

Salt and pepper to taste

Preparation:

- In a bowl, combine olive oil, lemon juice and zest, parsley, garlic, salt, and pepper.
- Add shrimp to the marinade and let sit for 30 minutes in the refrigerator.
- Preheat grill to high heat.
- Thread shrimp onto skewers and grill for about 3 minutes per side, or until opaque.

Benefits:

Shrimp is a great source of lean protein and omega-3 fatty acids, which are beneficial for heart health and cognitive function. The light marinade adds flavor without adding carbs.

6. Pork Tenderloin with Herb Rub

Preparation Time: 10 minutes

Cooking Time: 25 minutes

Ingredients:

1 pork tenderloin (about 1 lb)

2 tablespoons olive oil

1 tablespoon rosemary, minced

1 tablespoon thyme, minced

2 cloves garlic, minced

Salt and pepper to taste

Preparation:

- Preheat oven to 375°F (190°C).
- Rub the pork tenderloin with olive oil. Combine rosemary, thyme, garlic, salt, and pepper in a small bowl, and rub this mixture all over the pork.
- Place the pork on a roasting pan and roast for about 25 minutes, or until the internal temperature reaches 145°F (63°C).
- Let rest for 5 minutes before slicing.

Benefits:

Pork tenderloin is a lean source of protein that helps with muscle maintenance and repair. The herbs add flavor without extra carbs, supporting a low-carb diet.

7. Balsamic Roasted Brussels Sprouts

Preparation Time: 10 minutes

Cooking Time: 20 minutes

Ingredients:

2 cups Brussels sprouts, halved

2 tablespoons olive oil

2 tablespoons balsamic vinegar

Salt and pepper to taste

Preparation:

- Preheat oven to 400°F (200°C).
- Toss Brussels sprouts with olive oil, balsamic vinegar, salt, and pepper.
- Spread on a baking sheet and roast for 20 minutes, stirring halfway through, until caramelized and tender.

Benefits:

Brussels sprouts are high in fiber and vitamins C and K, which help support immune function and bone health. The low-carb profile fits well into a carb-cycling diet.

8. Creamy Tuscan Chicken

Preparation Time: 15 minutes

Cooking Time: 20 minutes

Ingredients:

2 boneless, skinless chicken breasts

1 tablespoon olive oil

1/2 cup sun-dried tomatoes, chopped

2 cloves garlic, minced

1 cup heavy cream

1/2 cup grated Parmesan cheese

1 cup spinach leaves

Salt and pepper to taste

Preparation:

- Heat olive oil in a skillet over medium heat. Add chicken breasts and cook until golden and nearly cooked through, about 7 minutes per side.
- Add garlic and sun-dried tomatoes to the skillet; cook for 2 minutes.
- Lower the heat, add heavy cream and Parmesan, and simmer until the sauce thickens.
- Stir in spinach and cook until wilted. Season with salt and pepper.

Benefits:

This dish is rich in protein and healthy fats, which are essential for muscle repair and satiety. The low-carb content helps with fat loss while providing a creamy, satisfying meal.

9. Spiced Lamb Kebabs

Preparation Time: 20 minutes (plus marinating)

Cooking Time: 10 minutes

Ingredients:

1 lb lamb, cut into cubes

2 tablespoons olive oil

1 teaspoon cumin

1 teaspoon coriander

1/2 teaspoon cinnamon

1/4 teaspoon allspice

Salt and pepper to taste

Preparation:

- In a bowl, mix olive oil, cumin, coriander, cinnamon, allspice, salt, and pepper.
- Add lamb cubes to the marinade and let sit for at least 2 hours in the refrigerator.
- Preheat grill to medium-high heat. Thread lamb onto skewers.
- Grill for about 10 minutes, turning occasionally, until cooked to desired doneness.

Benefits:

Lamb is a good source of high-quality protein and essential vitamins and minerals, supporting muscle growth and overall health. The spices enhance metabolism and provide antioxidant benefits.

10. Herb-Crusted Cod

Preparation Time: 10 minutes

Cooking Time: 15 minutes

Ingredients:

2 cod fillets (6 oz each)

1 tablespoon olive oil

1/4 cup almond flour

1 tablespoon chopped fresh parsley

1 teaspoon chopped fresh thyme

Salt and pepper to taste

Preparation:

- Preheat oven to 400°F (200°C).
- Brush cod fillets with olive oil. Mix almond flour, parsley, thyme, salt, and pepper in a bowl.
- Coat the cod evenly with the herb mixture.
- Place on a lined baking sheet and bake for 15 minutes, or until fish flakes easily with a fork.

Benefits:

Cod is a low-fat, high-protein fish that's also rich in omega-3 fatty acids, helping to support heart and brain health. The almond flour provides a gluten-free alternative to breadcrumbs, making this dish suitable for those on a gluten-free or low-carb diet.

11. Spicy Shrimp Avocado Salad

Preparation Time: 10 minutes

Cooking Time: 5 minutes

Ingredients:

1 lb shrimp, peeled and deveined

2 avocados, diced

1 cup cherry tomatoes, halved

1/2 cucumber, diced

1/4 cup red onion, finely chopped

1 jalapeño, seeded and finely chopped

Juice of 2 limes

2 tablespoons olive oil

Salt and pepper to taste

Fresh cilantro, chopped (for garnish)

Preparation:

- Heat olive oil in a skillet over medium-high heat.
- Add shrimp and cook until pink and opaque, about 2-3 minutes per side. Season with salt and pepper.
- In a large bowl, combine cooked shrimp, avocados, cherry tomatoes, cucumber, red onion, and jalapeño.
- Drizzle with lime juice, toss to combine.
- Garnish with fresh cilantro before serving.

Benefits:

Shrimp is a low-calorie protein source rich in selenium and vitamin B12. Avocados add healthy fats and fiber, promoting heart health and satiety.

12. Grilled Peach and Chicken Salad

Preparation Time: 15 minutes

Cooking Time: 10 minutes

Ingredients:

2 boneless, skinless chicken breasts

2 peaches, sliced into wedges

Mixed salad greens

1/4 cup crumbled feta cheese

1/4 cup balsamic vinaigrette

Preparation:

- Grill chicken breasts until fully cooked, about 5-7 minutes per side, then slice thinly.
- Grill peach wedges until char marks appear, about 2-3 minutes per side.
- Toss mixed greens with balsamic vinaigrette.
- Top greens with grilled chicken, grilled peaches, and feta cheese.

Benefits:

This salad offers a perfect blend of proteins, healthy fats, and carbohydrates. Peaches provide beneficial antioxidants and add a sweet flavor that complements the savory chicken.

13. Quinoa and Black Bean Salad

Preparation Time: 15 minutes

Cooking Time: 15 minutes

Ingredients:

1 cup quinoa

2 cups water

1 can black beans, drained and rinsed

1 red bell pepper, diced

1/4 cup finely chopped red onion

1/4 cup chopped fresh cilantro

Juice of 1 lime

2 tablespoons olive oil

Salt and pepper to taste

Preparation:

- Rinse quinoa under cold running water. Add to a pot with 2 cups of water. Bring to a boil, then cover and simmer for about 15 minutes or until water is absorbed.
- Let quinoa cool, then fluff with a fork.

- In a large bowl, combine cooled quinoa, black beans, red bell pepper, red onion, and cilantro.
- In a small bowl, whisk together lime juice, olive oil, salt, and pepper. Pour over the salad and toss to combine.

Benefits:

Quinoa is a complete protein source, containing all nine essential amino acids, making it exceptionally beneficial for vegetarians and vegans. Black beans add fiber and additional protein, supporting digestive health and energy levels.

14. Lemon Garlic Tilapia

Preparation Time: 5 minutes

Cooking Time: 10 minutes

Ingredients:

4 tilapia fillets

2 tablespoons butter

Juice of 1 lemon

2 garlic cloves, minced

Salt and pepper to taste

Fresh parsley, chopped (for garnish)

Preparation:

- Preheat oven to 400°F (200°C).
- Place tilapia fillets in a baking dish. Dot each fillet with butter, sprinkle with minced garlic, and drizzle with lemon juice. Season with salt and pepper.
- Bake in the preheated oven for about 10 minutes, or until fish flakes easily with a fork.
- Garnish with fresh parsley before serving.

Benefits:

Tilapia is a low-fat source of protein, making it ideal for a light meal that supports cardiovascular health. Lemon and garlic not only enhance the flavor but also provide vitamin C and have antibacterial properties.

Low-Carb Snacks and Smoothies

1. Cucumber Hummus Bites

Preparation Time: 5 minutes

Ingredients:

1 large cucumber, sliced into rounds

1/2 cup hummus

Paprika for sprinkling

Fresh parsley, chopped

Preparation:

- Top each cucumber round with a spoonful of hummus.
- Sprinkle with paprika, and garnish with chopped parsley.

Benefits:

Cucumbers are low in carbs and provide a refreshing crunch. Paired with hummus, they offer a good mix of fiber and protein.

2. Keto Berry Smoothie

Preparation Time: 5 minutes

Ingredients:

1/2 cup mixed berries (strawberries, blueberries)

1 cup unsweetened almond milk

1 tablespoon chia seeds

1 tablespoon MCT oil

Stevia to taste

Preparation:

- Blend all ingredients until smooth.

Benefits:

Berries provide antioxidants without excessive sugar, chia seeds add fiber, and MCT oil helps with ketone production, enhancing the low-carb benefits.

3. Almond Butter Celery Sticks

Preparation Time: 5 minutes

Ingredients:

2 stalks of celery, cut into 3-inch sticks

1/4 cup almond butter

1 tablespoon crushed almonds

Preparation:

- Spread almond butter on each celery stick, and sprinkle with crushed almonds.

Benefits:

Celery sticks are low in calories and carbs, while almond butter provides healthy fats and protein, making this a satisfying, crunchy snack.

4. Cheese and Walnut Stuffed Mushrooms

Preparation Time: 10 minutes

Cooking Time: 15 minutes

Ingredients:

6 large mushrooms, stems removed

1/2 cup cream cheese, softened

1/4 cup walnuts, chopped

1 garlic clove, minced

Salt and pepper to taste

Preparation:

- Preheat oven to 375°F (190°C).
- Mix cream cheese, walnuts, garlic, salt, and pepper in a bowl.
- Stuff each mushroom cap with the cheese mixture.
- Bake for 15 minutes until the mushrooms are tender.

Benefits:

Mushrooms are low in carbs and high in selenium and B vitamins, while cream cheese and walnuts provide fats and proteins.

5. Spinach and Feta Cheese Mini Quiches

Preparation Time: 10 minutes

Cooking Time: 20 minutes

Ingredients:

4 eggs, beaten

1/2 cup chopped spinach

1/4 cup feta cheese, crumbled

Salt and pepper to taste

Butter for greasing

Preparation:

- Preheat oven to 350°F (175°C). Grease a mini muffin pan with butter.
- Mix eggs, spinach, feta, salt, and pepper.
- Pour the mixture into the muffin pan cups.
- Bake for 20 minutes until set.

Benefits:

Spinach offers vitamins and minerals, and feta provides a good source of calcium and protein.

6. Spicy Tuna Salad Lettuce Wraps

Preparation Time: 10 minutes

Ingredients:

1 can (5 oz) tuna in water, drained

1/4 cup mayonnaise

1/2 teaspoon chili flakes

1 teaspoon lemon juice

Salt and pepper to taste

4 large lettuce leaves (such as romaine or iceberg)

Preparation:

- In a bowl, mix the tuna, mayonnaise, chili flakes, lemon juice, salt, and pepper.
- Spoon the tuna mixture into the center of each lettuce leaf and wrap.

Benefits:

Tuna is a great source of lean protein and omega-3 fatty acids, which are beneficial for heart health. Lettuce wraps are a low-carb alternative to bread, making this a perfect snack for a low-carb diet.

7. Greek Yogurt and Cucumber Dip

Preparation Time: 5 minutes

Ingredients:

1 cup Greek yogurt

1/2 cucumber, finely diced

1 tablespoon dill, chopped

1 garlic clove, minced

Salt and pepper to taste

Preparation:

- Combine all the ingredients in a bowl. Chill before serving.

Benefits:

Greek yogurt is high in protein and probiotics, which are good for digestive health. Cucumber adds freshness and hydration without many carbs.

8. Cheddar and Bacon Stuffed Mini Peppers

Preparation Time: 10 minutes

Cooking Time: 15 minutes

Ingredients:

6 mini bell peppers, halved and seeded

1/2 cup cheddar cheese, grated

3 slices of bacon, cooked and crumbled

Preparation:

- Preheat oven to 350°F (175°C).
- Place the halved peppers on a baking sheet.
- Fill each pepper half with cheese and top with crumbled bacon.
- Bake for 15 minutes until the peppers are tender and the cheese is melted.

Benefits:

Bell peppers are low in carbs and rich in vitamins A and C. The combination of cheddar and bacon provides a satisfying mix of fat and protein, making it a filling snack.

9. Avocado Chocolate Mousse

Preparation Time: 5 minutes

Ingredients:

1 ripe avocado

2 tablespoons cocoa powder

2 tablespoons almond milk

1 tablespoon honey or sweetener of choice

Preparation:

- Blend all ingredients until smooth in a food processor or blender.
- Chill before serving.

Benefits:

Avocado provides healthy fats that are essential for a low-carb diet. Cocoa powder is low in carbs and rich in antioxidants, offering a guilt-free way to satisfy a sweet craving.

Low-Carb Desserts

1. Almond Flour Chocolate Chip Cookies

Preparation Time: 15 minutes

Cooking Time: 12 minutes

Ingredients:

1 cup almond flour

1/4 cup coconut oil, melted

1/4 cup erythritol (or another keto-friendly sweetener)

1 egg

1/2 teaspoon baking powder

1/2 teaspoon vanilla extract

1/4 cup sugar-free chocolate chips

Preparation:

- Preheat the oven to 350°F (175°C).

- In a bowl, combine almond flour, baking powder, and erythritol.

- Mix in the egg, melted coconut oil, and vanilla extract until well combined.

- Fold in chocolate chips.

- Drop spoonfuls of the dough onto a baking sheet lined with parchment paper.

- Bake for 12 minutes or until edges are golden brown.

Benefits:

These cookies are rich in healthy fats and protein from almond flour and are low in carbs, making them a guilt-free treat.

2. Keto Lemon Bars

Preparation Time: 20 minutes

Cooking Time: 25 minutes

Ingredients:

For the crust:

1 cup almond flour

1/3 cup butter, melted

2 tablespoons erythritol

For the filling:

3 eggs

1/2 cup erythritol

1/2 cup lemon juice

2 tablespoons lemon zest

1/4 cup almond flour

Preparation:

- Preheat oven to 350°F (175°C).

- Mix almond flour, melted butter, and erythritol to form a dough. Press into the bottom of a prepared 8x8 inch baking dish.

- Bake the crust for 8 minutes.

- Whisk together the eggs, erythritol, lemon juice, zest, and almond flour. Pour over the baked crust.

- Bake for 17 minutes, or until set.

- Let cool before slicing into bars.

Benefits:

These lemon bars are refreshing and packed with vitamin C from the lemon, which hasa low glycemic index due to erythritol.

3. Coconut Flour Pancakes

Preparation Time: 10 minutes

Cooking Time: 15 minutes

Ingredients:

1/4 cup coconut flour

1/2 teaspoon baking powder

2 eggs

1/4 cup almond milk

1 tablespoon erythritol

1 teaspoon vanilla extract

Butter or oil for cooking

Preparation:

- Mix coconut flour and baking powder in a bowl.
- In another bowl, whisk eggs, almond milk, erythritol, and vanilla.
- Combine wet and dry ingredients until smooth.
- Heat butter in a skillet over medium heat. Pour batter to form small pancakes.
- Cook until bubbles form and edges are dry, then flip and cook for another minute.

Benefits:

Coconut flour is high in fiber and low in carbs, making these pancakes filling and suitable for a low-carb diet.

4. Strawberry Cheesecake Bites

Preparation Time: 20 minutes

Cooking Time: N/A

Ingredients:

1 cup strawberries, hulled

1/2 cup cream cheese, softened

1/4 cup powdered erythritol

1/2 teaspoon vanilla extract

Crushed almonds for coating

Preparation:

- Blend strawberries, cream cheese, erythritol,and vanilla extract until smooth.

- Shape the mixture into small balls and roll in crushed almonds.
- Chill in the refrigerator for 2 hours before serving.

Benefits:

These bites provide a good source of vitamin C and antioxidants from strawberries, combined with the creamy texture of cream cheese, making them a delightful low-carb treat.

5. Chocolate Peanut Butter Fat Bombs

Preparation Time: 15 minutes

Cooking Time: N/A

Ingredients:

1/2 cup coconut oil, melted

1/2 cup unsweetened peanut butter

1/4 cup unsweetened cocoa powder

2 tablespoons erythritol

Preparation:

- Mix melted coconut oil, peanut butter, cocoa powder, and erythritol until well combined.
- Pour the mixture into silicone molds or small cupcake liners.
- Freeze until solid, about 1 hour.

Benefits:

Rich in healthy fats and very low in carbs, these fat bombs are perfect for satisfying sweet cravings while maintaining ketosis.

6. Raspberry Almond Crumble

Preparation Time: 15 minutes

Cooking Time: 25 minutes

Ingredients:

1 cup fresh raspberries

1 cup almond flour

1/4 cup butter, chilled and diced

2 tablespoons erythritol

Preparation:

- Preheat oven to 350°F (175°C).
- Place raspberries in a small baking dish.
- In a bowl, combine almond flour, butter, and erythritol until crumbly.
- Sprinkle the crumble mixture over the raspberries.

- Bake for 25 minutes, or until the topping is golden brown.

Benefits:

Raspberries are high in fiber and vitamins, and almond flour provides a gluten-free, low-carb topping, making this a healthy and delicious dessert.

7. Vanilla Chia Pudding

Preparation Time: 5 minutes (plus 4 hours chilling time)

Cooking Time: N/A

Ingredients:

1/4 cup chia seeds

1 cup unsweetened almond milk

1 tablespoon erythritol

1 teaspoon vanilla extract

Preparation:

- Mix all ingredients in a bowl.
- Stir well and let sit for 5 minutes.
- Stir again, cover, and refrigerate for at least 4 hours or overnight.

Benefits:

Chia seeds are rich in omega-3 fatty acids, fibers, and proteins, making this pudding a superfood treat that helps with weight management and provides sustained energy.

8. Pumpkin Spice Muffins

Preparation Time: 15 minutes

Cooking Time: 20 minutes

Ingredients:

1 cup almond flour

1/2 cup pumpkin puree

2 eggs

1/4 cup erythritol

1 teaspoon pumpkin pie spice

1/2 teaspoon baking powder

Preparation:

- Preheat oven to 350°F (175°C).
- Mix all ingredients in a bowl until well combined.
- Divide batter into a greased muffin tin.

- Bake for 20 minutes or until a toothpick inserted comes out clean.

Benefits:

Pumpkin is low in calories but high in vitamins, particularly vitamin A, and the spices add flavor without adding carbs, making these muffins a perfect fall treat.

9. Lemon Poppy Seed Muffins

Preparation Time: 10 minutes

Cooking Time: 20 minutes

Ingredients:

1 cup almond flour

1/4 cup erythritol

2 tablespoons poppy seeds

1 teaspoon baking powder

1/4 teaspoon salt

3 eggs

1/4 cup melted butter

1/4 cup lemon juice

Zest of 1 lemon

Preparation:

- Preheat oven to 350°F (175°C).
- In a bowl, combine almond flour, erythritol, poppy seeds, baking powder, and salt.
- In another bowl, whisk together eggs, melted butter, lemon juice, and lemon zest.
- Mix the wet ingredients into the dry ingredients until well combined.
- Distribute the batter into a greased muffin tin.
- Bake for 20 minutes or until a toothpick inserted into the center comes out clean.

Benefits:

These muffins are not only low in carbs but also provide a good amount of healthy fats and protein. Lemon and poppy seeds add a refreshing flavor along with antioxidants and minerals.

Merry Lott

CHAPTER 7
HIGH-CARB RECIPES

High-Carb Breakfasts

1. Banana Oat Pancakes

Preparation Time: 10 minutes

Cooking Time: 10 minutes

Ingredients:

1 ripe banana

1 cup rolled oats

1 egg

1/2 cup low-fat milk

1 teaspoon baking powder

1/2 teaspoon vanilla extract

1 tablespoon honey

Butter or oil for cooking

Preparation:

- In a blender, combine the banana, rolled oats, egg, milk, baking powder, and vanilla extract. Blend until smooth.
- Heat a non-stick skillet over medium heat and add a little butter or oil.
- Pour about 1/4 cup of the batter for each pancake. Cook until bubbles form on the surface, then flip and cook until golden brown.
- Serve hot with a drizzle of honey.

Benefits:

These pancakes are a great source of complex carbohydrates and fiber from oats, providing sustained energy throughout the morning. Bananas add natural sweetness and potassium.

2. Sweet Potato Hash with Eggs

Preparation Time: 15 minutes

Cooking Time: 20 minutes

Ingredients:

2 medium sweet potatoes, peeled and diced

1 onion, chopped

1 red bell pepper, diced

2 cloves garlic, minced

4 eggs

2 tablespoons olive oil

Salt and pepper, to taste

Fresh parsley, chopped (for garnish)

Preparation:

- Heat olive oil in a large skillet over medium heat. Add the sweet potatoes, onion, and bell pepper. Cook until the vegetables are tender and beginning to brown, about 10 minutes.
- Add the garlic and cook for another 2 minutes.
- Make four wells in the hash and crack an egg into each. Cover the skillet and cook until eggs are set, about 8-10 minutes.
- Season with salt and pepper, garnish with parsley, and serve.

Benefits:

Sweet potatoes are high in vitamins A and C and provide a good source of complex carbs. This meal is balanced with protein from the eggs, keeping you full and energized.

3. Berry Quinoa Breakfast Bowl

Preparation Time: 5 minutes

Cooking Time: 15 minutes

Ingredients:

1 cup quinoa

2 cups water

1 cup mixed berries (fresh or frozen)

1/2 cup Greek yogurt

2 tablespoons honey

1/4 cup chopped nuts (e.g., almonds or walnuts)

Preparation:

- Rinse the quinoa under cold, running water. In a saucepan, bring water to a boil. Add quinoa, reduce heat to low, cover, and simmer for 15 minutes or until all water is absorbed.
- Divide the cooked quinoa into bowls. Top with berries, a dollop of Greek yogurt, a drizzle of honey, and a sprinkle of chopped nuts.

Benefits:

Quinoa provides a high protein content and all nine essential amino acids, making it an excellent plant-based protein source. Berries add antioxidants, and Greek yogurt provides calcium and probiotics.

4. Classic French Toast

Preparation Time: 10 minutes

Cooking Time: 10 minutes

Ingredients:

4 slices of whole grain bread

2 eggs

1/2 cup low-fat milk

1 teaspoon cinnamon

1 teaspoon vanilla extract

Maple syrup, for serving

Butter for cooking

Preparation:

- In a shallow dish, whisk together eggs, milk, cinnamon, and vanilla extract.
- Dip each slice of bread in the egg mixture, allowing it to soak on both sides.
- Heat a skillet over medium heat and add a little butter.
- Cook each slice until golden brown on both sides.
- Serve hot with maple syrup.

Benefits:

Whole grain bread provides a good source of fiber and complex carbohydrates. Eggs add protein, making this a balanced breakfast that will keep you satisfied.

5. Mango Coconut Overnight Oats

Preparation Time: 10 minutes

Cooking Time: 0 minutes (overnight chilling)

Ingredients:

1 cup rolled oats

1 cup coconut milk - 1 mango, peeled and diced

1 tablespoon chia seeds

2 tablespoons shredded coconut

1 tablespoon honey or maple syrup

Preparation:

- In a large bowl, mix the rolled oats, coconut milk, chia seeds, and honey or maple syrup.
- Divide the mixture into two jars or containers.
- Top with diced mango and shredded coconut.

- Cover and refrigerate overnight.

Benefits:

Mango provides essential vitamins and minerals, enhancing skin and immune health. Oats and chia seeds are excellent sources of fiber and omega-3 fatty acids, which are beneficial for heart health and digestion.

6. Cinnamon Apple Porridge

Preparation Time: 5 minutes

Cooking Time: 15 minutes

Ingredients:

1 cup steel-cut oats

2 cups water

1 apple, peeled and chopped

1 teaspoon cinnamon

1 tablespoon honey

1/2 cup almond milk

Preparation:

- In a saucepan, bring water to a boil. Add steel-cut oats and simmer on low for about 15 minutes, stirring occasionally.
- Halfway through cooking, add the chopped apple and cinnamon.
- Once the porridge is creamy and the oats are tender, remove from heat and stir in almond milk and honey.
- Serve warm.

Benefits:

Steel-cut oats are a hearty, high-fiber grain that helps manage blood sugar levels. Apples contribute additional fiber and vitamin C, while cinnamon offers anti-inflammatory properties.

7. Chocolate Banana Smoothie Bowl

Preparation Time: 10 minutes

Cooking Time: 0 minutes

Ingredients:

2 ripe bananas

1/4 cup rolled oats

2 tablespoons cocoa powder

1 cup almond milk

1 tablespoon honey

Toppings: sliced banana, granola, chia seeds

Preparation:

- In a blender, combine bananas, rolled oats, cocoa powder, almond milk, and honey. Blend until smooth.
- Pour into bowls and top with sliced banana, granola, and chia seeds.

Benefits:

Bananas are rich in potassium and magnesium, which help in muscle function and recovery. Cocoa powder adds antioxidants, and oats provide sustained energy.

8. Zucchini Bread Oatmeal

Preparation Time: 5 minutes

Cooking Time: 15 minutes

Ingredients:

1 cup rolled oats

2 cups water

1 small zucchini, grated

1 teaspoon cinnamon

2 tablespoons maple syrup

1/4 cup raisins

Preparation:

- In a saucepan, bring water to a boil. Add oats and grated zucchini and reduce to a simmer.
- Cook for about 10-15 minutes until the oats are soft.
- Stir in cinnamon, maple syrup, and raisins.
- Serve warm.

Benefits:

Zucchini is low in calories but high in essential nutrients like potassium and vitamin A. Oats provide a filling base, making this a satisfying and nutritious breakfast option.

9. Peanut Butter Jelly Overnight Oats

Preparation Time: 10 minutes

Cooking Time: 0 minutes (overnight chilling)

Ingredients:

1 cup rolled oats

1 cup almond milk

2 tablespoons peanut butter

2 tablespoons strawberry jam

1/2 banana, sliced

Preparation:

- In a jar, mix the rolled oats with almond milk.
- Add peanut butter and strawberry jam, and stir well.
- Top with sliced banana.
- Cover and refrigerate overnight.

Benefits:

Peanut butter provides protein and healthy fats, which are essential for muscle health and energy. Oats are a great source of carbohydrates for sustained energy.

10. Blueberry Bagel French Toast

Preparation Time: 10 minutes

Cooking Time: 10 minutes

Ingredients:

2 whole wheat bagels, sliced into halves

2 eggs

1/2 cup low-fat milk

1 teaspoon vanilla extract

1/2 cup fresh blueberries

1 tablespoon maple syrup

Butter for cooking

Preparation:

- In a shallow dish, whisk together the eggs, milk, and vanilla extract.
- Soak each bagel half in the egg mixture, ensuring both sides are coated.
- Heat a skillet over medium heat and add a small amount of butter.
- Place the soaked bagel halves in the skillet and cook until golden brown on each side, about 3-5 minutes per side.
- Serve the French toast warm, topped with fresh blueberries and a drizzle of maple syrup.

Benefits:

Whole wheat bagels provide a solid base of complex carbohydrates for energy. Blueberries are high in antioxidants and vitamins, promoting heart health and cognitive function. Eggs add a good source of protein, making this breakfast both balanced and nourishing.

High-Carb Lunches

1. Sweet Potato and Chickpea Buddha Bowl

Preparation Time: 10 minutes

Cooking Time: 30 minutes

Ingredients:

2 medium sweet potatoes, peeled and cubed

1 can chickpeas, drained and rinsed

1 avocado, sliced

2 cups spinach leaves

1 tablespoon olive oil

1 teaspoon smoked paprika

Salt and pepper to taste

2 tablespoons tahini

Juice of 1 lemon

Preparation:

- Preheat oven to 400°F (200°C). Toss sweet potatoes and chickpeas with olive oil, paprika, salt, and pepper. Spread on a baking sheet and roast for 30 minutes, stirring halfway through.
- Assemble the bowls with a base of spinach leaves, topped with roasted sweet potatoes and chickpeas, and sliced avocado.
- Drizzle tahini and lemon juice over the top before serving.

Benefits:

Sweet potatoes are a great source of complex carbohydrates and fiber. Chickpeas add protein and fiber, making this bowl filling and energizing.

2. Pasta Primavera

Preparation Time: 10 minutes

Cooking Time: 20 minutes

Ingredients:

200g whole wheat pasta

1 zucchini, sliced

1 carrot, sliced

1 bell pepper, sliced

1/2 cup peas

1/2 cup broccoli florets

2 tablespoons olive oil

2 garlic cloves, minced

Salt and pepper to taste

1/4 cup grated Parmesan cheese

Preparation:

- Cook the pasta according to package instructions until al dente. Drain and set aside.

- In a large pan, heat olive oil over medium heat. Add garlic, zucchini, carrot, bell pepper, peas, and broccoli. Sauté until vegetables are tender.

- Toss the cooked pasta with the vegetables. Season with salt and pepper, and sprinkle with Parmesan cheese before serving.

Benefits:

Whole wheat pasta provides sustained energy with its complex carbohydrates. The vegetables add vitamins and minerals, enhancing overall health and vitality.

3. Mango Chicken Wraps

Preparation Time: 15 minutes

Cooking Time: 10 minutes

Ingredients:

2 chicken breasts, cooked and sliced

2 whole wheat tortillas

1 mango, peeled and sliced

1 avocado, sliced

1/4 cup fresh cilantro, chopped

2 tablespoons Greek yogurt

Salt and pepper to taste

Preparation:

- Lay out the tortillas on a flat surface. Spread Greek yogurt over each tortilla.

- Down the center of each tortilla, layer chicken, mango, avocado, and cilantro.

- Season with salt and pepper, roll up the tortillas tightly, and serve.

Benefits:

The whole wheat tortillas provide carbs, while the chicken offers lean protein. Mango adds a sweet, refreshing burst of flavor and is rich in vitamins A and C.

4. Tuna and Sweet Corn Pasta Salad

Preparation Time: 10 minutes

Cooking Time: 10 minutes

Ingredients:

200g whole wheat pasta (e.g., fusilli or penne)

1 can tuna in water, drained

1 cup sweet corn

1 red bell pepper, diced

1/2 cucumber, diced

2 tablespoons mayonnaise

1 tablespoon mustard

Salt and pepper to taste

Preparation:

- Cook pasta according to package instructions until al dente, drain, and let cool.
- In a large bowl, mix the cooled pasta with tuna, sweet corn, bell pepper, and cucumber.
- In a small bowl, combine mayonnaise and mustard, then fold into the pasta salad. Season with salt and pepper.
- Chill before serving, or serve immediately.

Benefits:

Tuna provides high-quality protein and omega-3 fatty acids. Whole wheat pasta offers sustained energy, and the colorful vegetables supply essential vitamins and minerals.

5. Greek Orzo Salad

Preparation Time: 15 minutes

Cooking Time: 10 minutes

Ingredients:

1 cup orzo pasta

1 cup cherry tomatoes, halved

1 cucumber, diced

1/2 red onion, thinly sliced

1/4 cup Kalamata olives, halved

1/4 cup feta cheese, crumbled

2 tablespoons olive oil

Juice of 1 lemon

Salt and pepper to taste

1 teaspoon dried oregano

Preparation:

- Cook the orzo according to package instructions until al dente; drain and let cool.
- In a large bowl, combine the orzo, tomatoes, cucumber, onion, olives, and feta cheese.
- In a small bowl, whisk together olive oil, lemon juice, salt, pepper, and oregano. Pour over the salad and toss to coat evenly.
- Serve chilled or at room temperature.

Benefits:

Orzo is a light pasta that provides carbohydrates for energy. Feta cheese adds a creamy texture and calcium, while olives offer healthy fats.

6. BBQ Chicken Pizza

Preparation Time: 15 minutes

Cooking Time: 12 minutes

Ingredients:

1 pre-made whole wheat pizza crust

1/2 cup BBQ sauce

1 cooked chicken breast, shredded

1/2 red onion, thinly sliced

1 cup mozzarella cheese, shredded

2 green onions, chopped

Preparation:

- Preheat oven as directed by the pizza crust package.
- Spread BBQ sauce over the crust. Top with shredded chicken, red onion, and mozzarella cheese.
- Bake according to crust instructions until the cheese is bubbly and golden.
- Garnish with green onions before serving.

Benefits:

Whole wheat crust provides a fiber-rich base. Chicken is an excellent source of protein, and the BBQ sauce adds a tangy flavor that stimulates the metabolism.

7. Asian Noodle Salad with Peanut Sauce

Preparation Time: 15 minutes

Cooking Time: 5 minutes

Ingredients:

200g rice noodles

1 carrot, julienned

1 bell pepper, thinly sliced

1/2 cucumber, julienned

1/4 cup cilantro, chopped

1/4 cup peanuts, crushed

For the Peanut Sauce:

2 tablespoons peanut butter

2 tablespoons soy sauce

1 tablespoon honey

Juice of 1 lime

1 teaspoon chili flakes (optional)

Preparation:

- Cook rice noodles according to package instructions, then rinse under cold water and drain.
- In a large bowl, combine noodles, carrot, bell pepper, cucumber, and cilantro.
- In a small bowl, whisk together peanut butter, soy sauce, honey, lime juice, and chili flakes until smooth. Pour over the noodle salad and toss to coat.
- Sprinkle with crushed peanuts before serving.

Benefits:

Rice noodles are a gluten-free source of carbohydrates. The colorful vegetables are rich in vitamins, and the peanut sauce provides healthy fats and protein, making this salad a well-rounded, energizing meal.

8. Spinach and Ricotta Stuffed Shells

Preparation Time: 20 minutes

Cooking Time: 25 minutes

Ingredients:

16 jumbo pasta shells

1 cup ricotta cheese

1 cup spinach, cooked and squeezed dry

1/2 cup grated Parmesan cheese

1 egg

2 cups marinara sauce

1/2 cup shredded mozzarella cheese

Salt and pepper to taste

Preparation:

- Preheat the oven to 375°F (190°C).
- Cook pasta shells according to package instructions until al dente, drain, and set aside to cool.

- In a bowl, mix ricotta, spinach, Parmesan, egg, salt, and pepper.

- Spoon the filling into each pasta shell. Place filled shells in a baking dish.

- Pour marinara sauce over the shells and sprinkle with mozzarella.

- Bake for 25 minutes, or until the cheese is bubbly and golden.

Benefits:

This meal offers a good balance of carbohydrates from the shells and protein from the cheeses. Spinach provides iron and folate, making this a nutrient-dense dish.

9. Lemon Herb Couscous with Vegetables

Preparation Time: 10 minutes

Cooking Time: 15 minutes

Ingredients:

1 cup couscous

1 1/4 cups vegetable broth

1 zucchini, diced

1 bell pepper, diced

1/2 cup cherry tomatoes, halved

1/4 cup fresh herbs (parsley, cilantro, or basil), chopped

2 tablespoons olive oil

Juice and zest of 1 lemon

Salt and pepper to taste

Preparation:

- Bring vegetable broth to a boil in a pot. Add couscous, cover, and remove from heat. Let stand for 5 minutes.

- In a skillet, heat olive oil over medium heat. Sauté zucchini and bell pepper until tender.

- Fluff the couscous with a fork and mix in cooked vegetables, cherry tomatoes, herbs, lemon juice, and zest. Season with salt and pepper.

- Serve warm or at room temperature.

Benefits:

Couscous is a quick-cooking source of carbohydrates. Lemon adds a boost of vitamin C, and the fresh herbs provide antioxidants.

10. Sweet and Sour Tofu with Rice

Preparation Time: 15 minutes

Cooking Time: 20 minutes

Ingredients:

200g firm tofu, cubed

1 cup cooked white rice

1 bell pepper, cut into pieces

1 small onion, chopped

1/2 cup pineapple chunks

2 tablespoons vegetable oil

1/4 cup sweet and sour sauce

Salt and pepper to taste

Preparation:

- Heat oil in a pan over medium heat. Add tofu and fry until golden brown on all sides.
- Add the bell pepper and onion to the pan, cook until they are soft.
- Stir in pineapple chunks and sweet and sour sauce. Heat through.
- Serve the tofu mixture over cooked rice.

Benefits:

Tofu is a great source of protein and calcium. Rice provides energy-boosting carbohydrates, and pineapple offers digestive enzymes and vitamin C.

11. Mediterranean Farro Salad

Preparation Time: 10 minutes

Cooking Time: 30 minutes

Ingredients:

1 cup farro

3 cups water

1 cucumber, diced

1/2 cup sun-dried tomatoes, chopped

1/4 cup olives, chopped

1/4 cup feta cheese, crumbled

1/4 cup red onion, finely chopped

3 tablespoons olive oil

Juice of 1 lemon

1 teaspoon dried oregano

Salt and pepper to taste

Preparation:

- Rinse Farro under cold water. Bring water to a boil in a pot, add farro, reduce heat to low, cover, and simmer for about 30 minutes or until tender.

- Drain farro and let cool.

- In a large bowl, combine farro, cucumber, sun-dried tomatoes, olives, feta cheese, red onion, olive oil, lemon juice, and oregano. Toss everything together, and season with salt and pepper.

- Chill in the refrigerator before serving to blend the flavors.

Benefits:

Farro is rich in fiber and protein, making it an excellent base for salads. The additional ingredients like cucumber and tomatoes add freshness and vitamins, while feta cheese provides a creamy texture and a punch of flavor. This salad is perfect for a healthy, filling meal that's also great for heart health.

12. Grilled Vegetable and Hummus Wrap

Preparation Time: 10 minutes

Cooking Time: 10 minutes

Ingredients:

2 large whole wheat wraps

1/2 zucchini, sliced lengthwise

1/2 yellow squash, sliced lengthwise

1 red bell pepper, sliced

1/2 cup hummus

1 handful of spinach leaves

1 tablespoon olive oil

Salt and pepper to taste

Preparation:

- Preheat grill or grill pan to medium-high heat.

- Brush zucchini, squash, and bell pepper with olive oil; season with salt and pepper.

- Grill vegetables until tender and charred, about 3-4 minutes per side.

- Spread hummus on each wrap, place grilled vegetables and spinach leaves, and roll up tightly.

- Serve immediately, or wrap in foil for a portable lunch option.

Benefits:

This wrap offers a fantastic way to increase your intake of vegetables, providing vitamins, minerals, and fiber. Hummus adds protein and heart-healthy fats, making this a balanced, nutritious meal.

13. Pumpkin and Chickpea Curry

Preparation Time: 15 minutes

Cooking Time: 30 minutes

Ingredients:

1 tablespoon olive oil

1 onion, diced

2 cloves garlic, minced

1 tablespoon ginger, grated

1 tablespoon curry powder

2 cups pumpkin, cubed

1 can (15 oz) chickpeas, drained and rinsed

1 can (14 oz) coconut milk

1/2 cup vegetable broth

Salt and pepper to taste

Fresh cilantro for garnish

Preparation:

- Heat oil in a large skillet over medium heat. Add onion, garlic, and ginger; sauté until onion is translucent.
- Stir in curry powder and cook for another minute until fragrant.
- Add pumpkin, chickpeas, coconut milk, and vegetable broth. Bring to a simmer and cook until pumpkin is tender, about 20 minutes.
- Season with salt and pepper. Garnish with cilantro before serving.
- Serve hot with rice or naan.

Benefits:

Pumpkin is high in vitamins A and C, which are great for immune support. Chickpeas provide protein and fiber, making this curry a hearty, satisfying dish that's also good for digestive health.

14. Avocado Toast with Poached Egg

Preparation Time: 5 minutes

Cooking Time: 10 minutes

Ingredients:

2 slices of whole grain bread

1 ripe avocado

2 eggs

Salt and pepper to taste

Optional toppings: cherry tomatoes, radishes, arugula

Preparation:

- Toast the bread slices to your preference.

- Mash the avocado in a bowl and season with salt and pepper. Spread evenly on the toasted bread.

- Poach the eggs: bring a pot of water to a gentle simmer, add a splash of vinegar, and carefully drop the eggs into the water. Cook for about 3-4 minutes until the whites are set but yolks are still runny.

- Place a poached egg on each slice of avocado toast. Add additional toppings, if desired.

- Serve immediately with a sprinkle of salt and pepper.

Benefits:

Avocado is rich in healthy fats, particularly monounsaturated fat, which can help reduce bad cholesterol levels. Whole-grain bread provides fiber, while eggs offer a high-quality protein and a range of vitamins and minerals.

15. Baked Salmon with Dill and Lemon

Preparation Time: 5 minutes

Cooking Time: 20 minutes

Ingredients:

4 salmon fillets

1 lemon, thinly sliced

Fresh dill

Salt and pepper to taste

1 tablespoon olive oil

Preparation:

- Preheat oven to 375°F (190°C).

- Place salmon fillets on a baking sheet lined with parchment paper.

- Drizzle with olive oil, and season with salt and pepper.

- Place lemon slices and dill on top of each fillet.

- Bake in the preheated oven for about 15-20 minutes, or until salmon is cooked through and flakes easily with a fork.

Benefits:

Salmon is a great source of omega-3 fatty acids, which are essential for heart health and cognitive function. The addition of lemon not only adds a refreshing flavor but also provides vitamin C, enhancing iron absorption from the meal.

16. Vegetable Stir-Fry with Tofu

Preparation Time: 10 minutes

Cooking Time: 15 minutes

Ingredients:

200g firm tofu, cubed,

2 tablespoons soy sauce

1 tablespoon sesame oil

1 red bell pepper, sliced

1 green bell pepper, sliced

1 carrot, julienned

1 onion, sliced

2 cloves garlic, minced

1 tablespoon ginger, minced

2 tablespoons vegetable oil

Preparation:

- In a large pan, heat vegetable oil over medium-high heat.
- Add tofu and fry until golden brown on all sides. Remove from the pan and set aside.
- In the same pan, add more oil if needed, and sauté garlic, ginger, and onion until fragrant.
- Addbell peppers, carrot, and continue to stir-fry for a few minutes until vegetables are tender yet crisp.
- Return the tofu to the pan, add soy sauce and sesame oil, and stir well to combine all the ingredients.
- Serve hot, ideally over a bed of steamed rice or noodles.

Benefits:

Tofu is a good source of protein and contains all nine essential amino acids. It's also a valuable plant source of iron and calcium. The vegetables add fiber, vitamins, and antioxidants, making this dish a balanced and healthful choice.

17. Greek Yogurt Parfait with Mixed Berries and Granola

Preparation Time: 5 minutes

Cooking Time: 0 minutes

Ingredients:

1 cup Greek yogurt (plain or vanilla)

1/2 cup mixed berries (strawberries, blueberries, raspberries)

1/4 cup granola

Honey or agave syrup (optional)

Preparation:

- In a serving glass or bowl, layer half of the Greek yogurt.
- Add a layer of mixed berries.
- Sprinkle half of the granola over the berries.
- Repeat the layers with the remaining yogurt, berries, and granola.
- Drizzle with honey or agave syrup if desired.

Benefits:

Greek yogurt provides a high protein content that helps in muscle maintenance and satiety. Berries are rich in antioxidants and vitamins, while granola adds a crunchy texture and fiber, making this parfait a wholesome snack or breakfast option.

18. Spinach and Mushroom Omelette

Preparation Time: 5 minutes

Cooking Time: 10 minutes

Ingredients:

3 eggs

1/2 cup fresh spinach, chopped

1/4 cup mushrooms, sliced

1 tablespoon olive oil

Salt and pepper to taste

Optional: cheese (feta, cheddar, etc.)

Preparation:

- In a mixing bowl, beat the eggs with salt and pepper.
- Heat olive oil in a skillet over medium heat.
- Add mushrooms and sauté until they begin to brown.
- Add spinach and cook until wilted.
- Pour the beaten eggs over the vegetables in the skillet, covering them evenly.
- Cook until the eggs are set on the bottom, then fold the omelette in half and continue cooking until the eggs are fully set.
- Serve hot, optionally topped with your choice of cheese.

Benefits:

Eggs are a very good source of inexpensive, high-quality protein. More than half the protein of an egg is found in the egg white along with vitamin B2 and lower amounts of fat than the yolk. Spinach is rich in iron and mushrooms provide beneficial minerals, making this omelette a nutrient-dense meal option.

High-Carb Dinners

1. Teriyaki Chicken with Steamed Rice

Preparation Time: 10 minutes

Cooking Time: 20 minutes

Ingredients:

2 chicken breasts, diced

1 cup teriyaki sauce

1 tablespoon vegetable oil

2 cups cooked white rice

1 green onion, sliced for garnish

Sesame seeds for garnish

Preparation:

- Heat the oil in a pan over medium heat. Add the diced chicken and cook until browned.
- Pour the teriyaki sauce over the chicken and simmer for 10 minutes.
- Serve the chicken over steamed rice, garnished with green onions and sesame seeds.

Benefits:

This meal provides a high carbohydrate content from the rice, which is essential for energy replenishment, particularly after workouts. The chicken offers high-quality protein for muscle repair.

2. Sweet Potato and Black Bean Burritos

Preparation Time: 20 minutes

Cooking Time: 25 minutes

Ingredients:

2 large sweet potatoes, peeled and diced

1 can black beans, drained and rinsed

2 large wheat tortillas

1 avocado, sliced

1/2 cup shredded cheese

1 teaspoon cumin

Salt and pepper to taste

Preparation:

- Boil or steam the sweet potatoes until tender.
- Mash the sweet potatoes and mix with cumin, salt, and pepper.
- Warm the tortillas. Spread the sweet potato mixture onto each tortilla.

- Top with black beans, avocado slices, and shredded cheese.
- Roll up the tortillas and serve.

Benefits:

Sweet potatoes are an excellent source of carbohydrates and fiber. Black beans add protein and fiber, making this a balanced, energy-boosting meal.

3. Quinoa Salad with Mango and Black Beans

Preparation Time: 15 minutes

Cooking Time: 15 minutes

Ingredients:

1 cup quinoa

2 cups water

1 mango, peeled and diced

1 can black beans, drained and rinsed

1 red bell pepper, diced

Juice of 1 lime

1 tablespoon olive oil

1/4 cup chopped cilantro

Salt to taste

Preparation:

- Rinse quinoa under cold running water. In a saucepan, bring water to a boil. Add quinoa, reduce heat to low, cover, and simmer for 15 minutes.
- Fluff the cooked quinoa with a fork and allow it to cool.
- In a large bowl, combine the quinoa, mango, black beans, and red bell pepper.
- Whisk together lime juice, olive oil, and salt. Pour over the salad and toss to coat.
- Stir in chopped cilantro before serving.

Benefits:

Quinoa is a complete protein, complemented by high-fiber black beans and mango, which adds a rich source of vitamins A and C.

4. Risotto with Mushrooms and Peas

Preparation Time: 10 minutes

Cooking Time: 30 minutes

Ingredients:

1 cup Arborio rice

1/2 cup fresh peas

1 cupmushrooms, sliced

4 cups vegetable broth

1 onion, finely chopped

2 cloves garlic, minced

1/4 cup white wine (optional)

2 tablespoons olive oil

1/4 cup grated Parmesan cheese

Salt and pepper to taste

Preparation:

- In a saucepan, heat the vegetable broth over medium heat.
- In another pan, heat olive oil over medium heat. Add onion and garlic, and sauté until translucent.
- Add Arborio rice to the pan with onions and stir to coat with oil.
- Pour in the white wine, if using, and let it evaporate.
- Add the hot broth one ladle at a time, stirring continuously, until the rice absorbs the liquid before adding more.
- When the rice is halfway done, add the mushrooms and peas.
- Continue to add broth and stir until the rice is creamy and al dente.
- Remove from heat, stir in the Parmesan cheese, and season with salt and pepper.

Benefits:

This dish is rich in carbohydrates and provides a good source of vegetable protein from peas. The mushrooms offer additional nutrients and fiber, making it a hearty, satisfying meal.

5. Chickpea and Spinach Curry

Preparation Time: 10 minutes

Cooking Time: 20 minutes

Ingredients:

1 can chickpeas, drained and rinsed

200g fresh spinach leaves

1 onion, chopped

2 cloves garlic, minced

1 tablespoon curry powder

1 can coconut milk

2 tablespoons oil

Salt to taste

Preparation:

- Heat oil in a pan over medium heat. Add onion and garlic, sauté until soft.
- Stir in curry powder and cook for another minute.
- Add chickpeas and coconut milk, bring to a simmer.
- Add spinach and cook until wilted.
- Season with salt, and let the curry simmer until thickened.

Benefits:

Chickpeas are an excellent source of carbohydrates and protein. Spinach adds fiber, vitamins, and minerals. This curry is great for a comforting, nutrient-dense dinner.

6. Baked Ziti with Ricotta and Marinara Sauce

Preparation Time: 15 minutes

Cooking Time: 25 minutes

Ingredients:

200g ziti pasta

1 cup ricotta cheese

2 cups marinara sauce

1/2 cup mozzarella cheese, shredded

2 tablespoons fresh basil, chopped

Salt and pepper to taste

Preparation:

- Preheat oven to 375°F (190°C).
- Cook pasta according to package instructions until al dente. Drain.
- In a mixing bowl, combine cooked pasta, ricotta cheese, and marinara sauce. Season with salt and pepper.
- Transfer to a baking dish and top with shredded mozzarella.
- Bake for 20-25 minutes, or until the cheese is bubbly and golden.
- Garnish with fresh basil before serving.

Benefits:

Pasta is a good source of energy-providing carbohydrates. Ricotta and mozzarella cheese add calcium and protein to this comforting dish.

7. Vegetable Stir-Fry with Brown Rice

Preparation Time: 10 minutes

Cooking Time: 20 minutes

Ingredients:

1 cup brown rice

2 cups water

1 tablespoon sesame oil

1 red bell pepper, sliced

1 carrot, sliced

1 cup broccoli florets

1/2 cup snap peas

2 tablespoons soy sauce

1 teaspoon ginger, grated

1 garlic clove, minced

Preparation:

- Cook brown rice with water according to package instructions.
- Heat sesame oil in a large skillet or wok. Add ginger and garlic, sauté for a minute.
- Add all vegetables and stir-fry until tender-crisp.
- Stir in soy sauce and cook for another minute.
- Serve the vegetable stir-fry over cooked brown rice.

Benefits:

Brown rice provides a wholesome source of carbohydrates. The variety of vegetables offers essential vitamins, minerals, and antioxidants, making this a balanced and nutritious meal.

8. Lemon Herb Salmon with Garlic Potatoes

Preparation Time: 10 minutes

Cooking Time: 25 minutes

Ingredients:

2 salmon fillets

2 tablespoons olive oil

4 cloves garlic, minced

Juice and zest of 1 lemon

1 tablespoon fresh dill, chopped

1 tablespoon fresh parsley, chopped

2 large potatoes, diced

Salt and pepper to taste

Preparation:

- Preheat your oven to 400°F (200°C).

- Toss the diced potatoes with 1 tablespoon olive oil, half of the minced garlic, salt, and pepper. Spread on a baking sheet and bake for 20 minutes, until golden and crisp.

- Meanwhile, mix the remaining olive oil, garlic, lemon juice and zest, dill, and parsley in a bowl.

- Place salmon fillets on a lined baking tray. Spoon the lemon herb mixture over the salmon.

- When potatoes are nearly done, add the salmon to the oven and bake for 12-15 minutes, or until cooked through.

- Serve the salmon with the crispy garlic potatoes.

Benefits:

Salmon is rich in omega-3 fatty acids, which are essential for heart health and brain function. Potatoes provide a high-carb source for sustained energy. This dish combines healthy fats, proteins, and carbs for a well-balanced meal.

9. Butternut Squash Risotto

Preparation Time: 15 minutes

Cooking Time: 30 minutes

Ingredients:

1 small butternut squash, peeled and diced

1 cup Arborio rice

4 cups vegetable stock, warm

1 onion, finely chopped

2 cloves garlic, minced

1/2 cup white wine (optional)

1/4 cup grated Parmesan cheese

2 tablespoons olive oil

Salt and pepper to taste

Preparation:

- Heat olive oil in a large pan over medium heat. Add onion and garlic, sauté until translucent.

- Add the Arborio rice and stir for a few minutes until the edges become slightly transparent.

- Pour in the white wine, if using, and let it evaporate.

- Add a ladle of warm vegetable stock and the diced butternut squash. Stir continuously until the liquid is absorbed.

- Continue adding stock one ladle at a time, allowing each addition to be absorbed before adding the next, until the rice is creamy and al dente.

- Stir in the Parmesan cheese, season with salt and pepper, and serve warm.

Benefits:

Butternut squash is a good source of vitamins A and C, fiber, and antioxidants. Combined with rice, it makes for a hearty, comforting dish that is also nutritious, providing a solid base of carbohydrates for energy.

10. Black Bean and Corn Quesadillas

Preparation Time: 10 minutes

Cooking Time: 10 minutes

Ingredients:

4 large flour tortillas

1 can black beans, drained and rinsed

1 cup corn kernels, fresh or frozen

1/2 cup shredded cheddar cheese

1/2 teaspoon chili powder

1 avocado, sliced

1/2 cup salsa

1 tablespoon vegetable oil

Preparation:

- Heat a non-stick pan over medium heat and brush with a little vegetable oil.
- Place a tortilla in the pan, On one half of the tortilla, spread a layer of black beans and corn. Sprinkle with chili powder and cheese.
- Fold the tortilla over to cover the filling. Cook for about 2-3 minutes on each side until golden and the cheese melts.
- Repeat with the remaining tortillas.
- Serve with slices of avocado and salsa on the side.

Benefits:

Black beans and corn together provide a high-carb, high-fiber content that helps maintain good digestive health and sustained energy levels. Cheese adds calcium and protein, making this an easy-to-make, balanced meal.

11. Creamy Tomato Pasta

Preparation Time: 5 minutes

Cooking Time: 15 minutes

Ingredients:

200g penne pasta

1 cup heavy cream

1 cup tomato sauce

1 garlic clove, minced

2tablespoons olive oil

1/4 cup grated Parmesan cheese

Salt and pepper to taste

Fresh basil for garnish

Preparation:

- Cook the penne pasta according to the package instructions until al dente. Drain and set aside.
- In the same pot, heat olive oil over medium heat. Add minced garlic and sauté until fragrant.
- Pour in the tomato sauce and heavy cream. Stir to combine, and bring to a simmer.
- Add the cooked pasta back into the pot, tossing to coat evenly with the sauce.
- Cook for an additional 2-3 minutes until everything is heated through.
- Season with salt and pepper. Serve hot, sprinkled with grated Parmesan and fresh basil leaves.

Benefits:

This dish is comforting and satisfying, providing a good balance of carbohydrates from the pasta and fats from the cream. Tomatoes offer vitamin C and other antioxidants, while the addition of Parmesan provides a tasty source of calcium and protein.

12. Vegetable Stir-Fry with Tofu

Preparation Time: 10 minutes

Cooking Time: 10 minutes

Ingredients:

1 block firm tofu, cubed

2 cups mixed vegetables (broccoli, bell peppers, carrots)

2 tablespoons soy sauce

1 tablespoon sesame oil

1 teaspoon ginger, grated

2 cloves garlic, minced

1 tablespoon cornstarch

1/4 cup water

Preparation:

- Heat sesame oil in a large skillet or wok over medium-high heat.
- Add garlic and ginger, and sauté for about 1 minute.
- Add the mixed vegetables and stir-fry for about 5 minutes, or until they begin to soften.
- In a small bowl, mix the cornstarch with water and soy sauce to create a slurry.

- Add the tofu to the skillet along with the soy sauce mixture. Cook, stirring frequently, until the sauce thickens and tofu is heated through, about 5 minutes.
- Serve hot.

Benefits:

Tofu is a good source of protein and contains all nine essential amino acids. It's also a valuable plant source of iron and calcium. The vegetables add fiber, vitamins, and minerals, making this a nutrient-dense meal that's also vegan-friendly.

13. Thai Green Curry with Chicken

Preparation Time: 15 minutes

Cooking Time: 20 minutes

Ingredients:

1 lb chicken breast, cut into bite-sized pieces

2 tablespoons green curry paste

1 can (14 oz) coconut milk

1 cup bamboo shoots, drained

1 bell pepper, sliced

1 zucchini, sliced

1 tablespoon fish sauce

1 teaspoon sugar

1/2 cup fresh basil leaves

2 tablespoons vegetable oil

Preparation:

- Heat the oil in a large skillet over medium heat. Add the green curry paste and sauté for about 1 minute until fragrant.
- Add the chicken and cook until it's no longer pink.
- Pour in the coconut milk, bring to a simmer.
- Add bamboo shoots, bell pepper, and zucchini. Simmer for about 10 minutes or until vegetables are tender.
- Stir in fish sauce and sugar. Adjust seasoning as needed.
- Just before serving, stir in fresh basil leaves.
- Serve hot over rice.

Benefits:

This dish is rich in protein from chicken and contains a variety of vegetables, which provide essential vitamins and minerals. Coconut milk adds a creamy texture and supplies healthy fats.

Merry Lott

14. Shrimp and Asparagus Risotto

Preparation Time: 10 minutes

Cooking Time: 30 minutes

Ingredients:

1 lb shrimp, peeled and deveined

1 bunch asparagus, trimmed and cut into pieces

1 cup Arborio rice

4 cups chicken or vegetable broth, warm

1 onion, finely chopped

1/2 cup white wine (optional)

1/4 cup grated Parmesan cheese

2 tablespoons of olive oil

Salt and pepper to taste

Preparation:

- In a large skillet, heat 1 tablespoon of olive oil over medium heat. Add the onion and cook until translucent.
- Add the Arborio rice and stir for a few minutes until the grains are well-coated with oil and slightly toasted.
- Pour in the white wine (if using) and let it evaporate.
- Gradually add the warm broth, one cup at a time, stirring constantly. Wait until each addition is almost fully absorbed before adding the next.
- Halfway through, add the asparagus. Continue to add broth and stir.
- When the rice is tender and creamy, add the shrimp. Cook until the shrimp are pink and cooked through.
- Stir in the Parmesan cheese, add salt and pepper to taste, and drizzle with the remaining olive oil. Serve hot.

Benefits:

This dish provides a good balance of carbohydrates from the rice and high-quality protein from the shrimp. Asparagus is rich in fiber, folate, and vitamins A, C, and K.

15. Quinoa Salad with Roasted Sweet Potatoes

Preparation Time: 15 minutes

Cooking Time: 25 minutes

Ingredients:

1 cup quinoa

2 sweet potatoes, peeled and cubed

1 red bell pepper, diced

1/4 cup dried cranberries

1/4 cup chopped walnuts

1/4 cup feta cheese, crumbled

3 tablespoons olive oil

2 tablespoons balsamic vinegar

Salt and pepper to taste

Preparation:

- Preheat the oven to 400°F (200°C). Toss sweet potatoes with 1 tablespoon of olive oil, salt, and pepper. Roast for about 20-25 minutes until tender.

- Meanwhile, cook the quinoa according to package instructions.

- In a large bowl, combine cooked quinoa, roasted sweet potatoes, red bell pepper, dried cranberries, and walnuts.

- Whisk together the remaining olive oil and balsamic vinegar, then pour over the salad. Toss to coat.

- Sprinkle with feta cheese before serving.

Benefits:

Quinoa is a complete protein source, which is rare for plant-based foods. It's also high in fiber and iron. Sweet potatoes are an excellent source of vitamin A and C, while walnuts provide healthy fats.

16. Mediterranean Grilled Chicken Salad

Preparation Time: 20 minutes

Cooking Time: 10 minutes

Ingredients:

2 boneless, skinless chicken breasts

1 bag mixed greens (lettuce, spinach, arugula)

1 cucumber, sliced

1 cup cherry tomatoes, halved

1/4 cup sliced olives

1/4 cup crumbled feta cheese

1/4 cup red onion, thinly sliced

2 tablespoons olive oil

2 tablespoons lemon juice

1 teaspoon dried oregano

Salt and pepper to taste

Preparation:

- Preheat grill to medium-high heat. Season chicken breasts with salt, pepper, and oregano.

- Grill chicken for about 5 minutes on each side or until fully cooked. Let it rest for a few minutes, then slice thinly.
- In a large bowl, combine mixed greens, cucumber, cherry tomatoes, olives, and red onion.
- In a small bowl, whisk together olive oil and lemon juice, then drizzle over the salad.
- Add the grilled chicken slices and sprinkle with feta cheese.
- Toss everything together and serve immediately.

Benefits:

This salad combines lean protein from the chicken with a variety of vegetables, offering a rich array of nutrients, including vitamins, minerals, and antioxidants. Olive oil and feta provide healthy fats that are good for heart health.

High-Carb Snacks and Smoothies

1. Banana Berry Smoothie

Preparation Time: 5 minutes

Ingredients:

2 ripe bananas

1 cup mixed berries (strawberries, blueberries, raspberries)

1 cup orange juice

1/2 cup Greek yogurt

1 tablespoon honey

Preparation:

- Combine all ingredients in a blender.
- Blend until smooth.

Benefits:

This smoothie is high in carbohydrates and antioxidants, making it perfect for energy replenishment post-exercise. Greek yogurt provides protein to aid in muscle recovery.

2. Oatmeal Raisin Energy Balls

Preparation Time: 15 minutes

Ingredients:

1 cup rolled oats

1/2 cup peanut butter

1/3 cup honey

1/2 cup raisins

1 teaspoon vanilla extract

Preparation:

- Mix all ingredients in a bowl until well combined.
- Roll into small balls and refrigerate for at least 1 hour before serving.

Benefits:

Packed with healthy fats from peanut butter and fiber from oats, these energy balls provide a quick, high-carb snack ideal for energy boosts before workouts.

3. Sweet Potato and Black Bean Burrito

Preparation Time: 10 minutes

Cooking Time: 20 minutes

Ingredients:

2 medium sweet potatoes, peeled and diced

1 can black beans, drained and rinsed

4 whole wheat tortillas

1 avocado, sliced

1/2 cup salsa

1 teaspoon cumin

Salt and pepper to taste

Preparation:

- Boil or steam sweet potatoes until soft.
- In a bowl, mix sweet potatoes, black beans, cumin, salt, and pepper.
- Divide the mixture among tortillas and top with avocado slices and salsa.
- Roll up the tortillas and serve.

Benefits:

This burrito is a balanced meal with high carbs from sweet potatoes and fiber-rich black beans, enhancing muscle glycogen replenishment.

4. Mango Chia Pudding

Preparation Time: 10 minutes (plus chilling)

Ingredients:

1 ripe mango, peeled and chopped

2 cups almond milk

1/2 cup chia seeds

1 tablespoon maple syrup

Preparation:

- Blend mango and almond milk until smooth.
- Pour into a bowl and add chia seeds and maple syrup.
- Stir well and refrigerate overnight or at least 4 hours.

Benefits:

Mango chia pudding is rich in omega-3 fatty acids from chia seeds and high in carbohydrates, ideal for starting the day with sustained energy.

5. Apple Cinnamon Quinoa Bites

Preparation Time: 15 minutes

Cooking Time: 20 minutes

Ingredients:

1 cup cooked quinoa

1 apple, grated

2 tablespoons honey

1 teaspoon cinnamon

1/2 cup rolled oats

Preparation:

- Preheat oven to 350°F (175°C).
- Combine all the ingredients in a bowl.
- Form into small balls and place on a baking sheet.
- Bake for 20 minutes.

Benefits:

These bites are a great source of complex carbohydrates and fiber, making them a perfect snack for sustained energy release.

6. Peanut Butter Banana Toast

Preparation Time: 5 minutes

Ingredients:

2 slices whole grain bread

1 large banana, sliced

2 tablespoons peanut butter

Preparation:

- Toast the bread slices.
- Spread peanut butter on each slice.

- Top with banana slices.

Benefits:

Combining whole grains with the natural sugars from bananas and protein from peanut butter, this snack offers a balanced approach to fueling up.

7. Yogurt and Fruit Parfait

Preparation Time: 10 minutes

Ingredients:

1 cup Greek yogurt

1/2 cup granola

1/2 cup mixed fresh fruit (berries, kiwi, mango)

Preparation:

- Layer Greek yogurt, granola, and mixed fruit in a tall glass.
- Repeat the layers until all ingredients are used.

Benefits:

Rich in high-quality carbs and proteins, this parfait is great for recovery and provides probiotics for digestive health.

8. Tropical Green Smoothie

Preparation Time: 5 minutes

Ingredients:

1 cup spinach

1 cup coconut water

1 banana

1/2 cup pineapple chunks

1/2 cup mango chunks

Preparation:

- Combine all ingredients in a blender.
- Blend until smooth.

Benefits:

This smoothie is loaded with vitamins and high in carbs, perfect for hydration and energy before intense workouts.

9. Cinnamon Apple Chips

Preparation Time: 10 minutes

Cooking Time: 2 hours

Ingredients:

2 apples, thinly sliced

1 teaspoon cinnamon

Preparation:

- Preheat oven to 200°F (95°C).
- Arrange apple slices on a baking sheet and sprinkle with cinnamon.
- Bake for 2 hours, flipping halfway through, until crispy.

Benefits:

A healthy, high-carb snack that is naturally sweet and perfect for a quick energy boost.

10. Blueberry Oatmeal Smoothie

Preparation Time: 5 minutes

Ingredients:

1 cup fresh blueberries

1/2 cup rolled oats

1 banana

1 cup almond milk

1 tablespoon honey

Preparation:

- Blend all ingredients until smooth.

Benefits:

This smoothie combines antioxidants from blueberries with the sustaining energy of oats, making it ideal for fueling up pre-workout.

High-Carb Desserts

1. Chocolate Banana Bread

Preparation Time: 15 minutes

Cooking Time: 50 minutes

Ingredients:

2 ripe bananas, mashed

1 cup all-purpose flour

1/2 cup cocoa powder

3/4 cup sugar

1/2 cup unsalted butter, melted

2 eggs

1 teaspoon baking powder

1 teaspoon vanilla extract

1/2 teaspoon salt

1/2 cup chocolate chips

Preparation:

- Preheat oven to 350°F (175°C). Grease a loaf pan.
- In a bowl, combine flour, cocoa powder, baking powder, and salt.
- In another bowl, mix mashed bananas, melted butter, sugar, eggs, and vanilla.
- Combine the wet and dry ingredients, then fold in chocolate chips.
- Pour batter into the prepared pan and bake for 50 minutes.

Benefits:

Provides a high-carb, energy-rich treat with the mood-lifting properties of chocolate. Perfect for post-workout recovery.

2. Peach Cobbler

Preparation Time: 20 minutes

Cooking Time: 30 minutes

Ingredients:

4 cups sliced peaches

1 cup all-purpose flour

1 cup sugar

1/2 cup unsalted butter, melted

1 teaspoon baking powder

1/4 teaspoon salt

1/2 cup milk

1 teaspoon cinnamon

Preparation:

- Preheat oven to 375°F (190°C).
- Spread peaches in a baking dish.
- In a bowl, mix flour, sugar, baking powder, and salt. Stir in milk and melted butter to form a batter.
- Pour batter over peaches and sprinkle with cinnamon.

- Bake for 30 minutes until golden.

Benefits:

Peaches provide natural sugars and fiber, while the dessert's high carbohydrate content helps replenish glycogen stores.

3. Maple Oatmeal Cookies

Preparation Time: 15 minutes

Cooking Time: 15 minutes

Ingredients:

1 cup rolled oats

3/4 cup all-purpose flour

1/2 cup maple syrup

1/2 cup unsalted butter, softened

1 egg

1/2 teaspoon baking soda

1/2 teaspoon cinnamon

1/4 teaspoon salt

Preparation:

- Preheat oven to 350°F (175°C). Line a baking sheet with parchment paper.
- In a bowl, combine oats, flour, baking soda, cinnamon, and salt.
- In another bowl, cream together butter and maple syrup until smooth. Beat in the egg.
- Gradually mix in the dry ingredients.
- Drop spoonfuls of the dough onto the prepared sheet, and bake for 15 minutes.

Benefits:

It offers a good mix of carbs and fats, perfect for a quick energy boost. Maple syrup provides a natural sweetness.

4. Rice Pudding

Preparation Time: 5 minutes

Cooking Time: 25 minutes

Ingredients:

1 cup cooked white rice

1 1/2 cups milk

1/3 cup sugar

1/4 teaspoon salt

1/2 teaspoon vanilla extract

1/4 teaspoon cinnamon

1/4 cup raisins

Preparation:

- In a saucepan, combine all ingredients except vanilla and cinnamon.
- Cook over medium heat, stirring until thickened (about 25 minutes).
- Remove from heat and stir in vanilla and cinnamon.

Benefits:

Rice pudding is a comforting, high-carb dessert that can help restore glycogen levels efficiently.

5. Lemon Bars

Preparation Time: 20 minutes

Cooking Time: 35 minutes

Ingredients:

For the crust:

1 cup all-purpose flour

1/4 cup sugar

1/2 cup unsalted butter, softened

For the filling:

2 eggs

1 cup sugar

2 tablespoons all-purpose flour

1/4 cup lemon juice

1 tablespoon lemon zest

Preparation:

- Preheat oven to 350°F (175°C). Line an 8-inch square baking dish with parchment paper.
- For the crust, combine flour, sugar, and butter until crumbly. Press into the bottom of the prepared dish. Bake for 15 minutes.
- For the filling, whisk together eggs, sugar, flour, lemon juice, and lemon zest until smooth. Pour over the baked crust.
- Bake for an additional 20 minutes, until the filling is set. Cool before slicing.

Benefits:

Lemon bars offer a refreshing taste and a good balance of carbohydrates, making them ideal for an energy boost and aiding in muscle recovery.

6. Sweet Potato Pie

Preparation Time: 30 minutes

Cooking Time: 55 minutes

Ingredients:

1 large sweet potato, peeled and cubed

1/2 cup sugar

1/2 cup milk

1/4 cup butter, softened

2 eggs

1 teaspoon vanilla extract

1/2 teaspoon ground cinnamon

1/4 teaspoon ground nutmeg

1 unbaked pie crust

Preparation:

- Boil sweet potato until soft, about 20 minutes; drain and mash.
- Mix mashed sweet potato with sugar, milk, butter, eggs, vanilla, cinnamon, and nutmeg until smooth.
- Pour into the unbaked pie crust.
- Bake at 350°F (175°C) for 35-40 minutes.

Benefits:

Sweet potatoes are high in carbohydrates and rich in vitamins, making this pie a nutritious choice for energy recovery.

7. Apple Crisp

Preparation Time: 15 minutes

Cooking Time: 45 minutes

Ingredients:

4 apples, peeled, cored, and sliced

3/4 cup brown sugar

1/2 cup all-purpose flour

1/2 cup rolled oats

1/3 cup butter, softened

1 teaspoon cinnamon

1/4 teaspoon nutmeg

Preparation:

- Preheat oven to 350°F (175°C).

- Place apple slices in a baking dish.

- In a bowl, mix brown sugar, flour, oats, butter, cinnamon, and nutmeg until crumbly. Sprinkle over apples.

- Bake for 45 minutes until topping is golden and apples are tender.

Benefits:

Apples provide natural sugars and dietary fiber, while oats are a sustaining source of carbohydrates.

8. Berry Trifle

Preparation Time: 30 minutes

Cooking Time: No cooking required

Ingredients:

2 cups mixed berries (strawberries, blueberries, raspberries)

1/2 cup sugar

2 cups vanilla pudding

1 cup whipped cream

2 cups cubed pound cake

Preparation:

- In a large bowl, toss berries with sugar.

- In a trifle dish, layer half of the cubed pound cake, topped with half of the berries and half of the vanilla pudding. Repeat layers.

- Top with whipped cream.

Benefits:

Berries are loaded with antioxidants, while the high-carb content of pound cake and pudding provides energy.

9. Chocolate Chip Pancake Syrup Cake

Preparation Time: 10 minutes

Cooking Time: 20 minutes

Ingredients:

1 cup pancake mix

1/2 cup milk

1 egg

1/2 cup chocolate chips

1/2 cup maple syrup

Merry Lott

Preparation:
- Preheat oven to 350°F (175°C).
- In a bowl, mix pancake mix, milk, and egg until smooth. Stir in chocolate chips.
- Pour into a greased 8-inch cake pan. Drizzle maple syrup over the top.
- Bake for 20 minutes.

Benefits:

A fun twist on traditional pancakes, offering a high carbohydrate load with the added sweetness of maple syrup.

10. Mango Coconut Rice Dessert

Preparation Time: 10 minutes

Cooking Time: 20 minutes

Ingredients:

1 cup cooked jasmine rice

1 cup coconut milk

1/2 cup sugar

1 ripe mango, peeled and diced

1/4 cup toasted coconut flakes

1 tsp vanilla extract

Pinch of salt

Preparation:
- In a medium saucepan, combine the cooked jasmine rice, coconut milk, and sugar. Add a pinch of salt to enhance the flavors.
- Cook over medium heat, stirring continuously, until the mixture thickens slightly, which should take about 15-20 minutes.
- Remove from heat and stir in vanilla extract. Allow the mixture to cool slightly; it will thicken further as it cools.
- Spoon the warm rice into serving dishes. Top each serving with diced mango and sprinkle with toasted coconut flakes for added texture and flavor.

Benefits:

This dessert not only satisfies sweet cravings but also provides a good source of energy from the carbohydrates in the rice and mango. Coconut milk adds a creamy texture and supplies medium-chain triglycerides (MCTs), which are known for their energy-boosting properties. Mango is a rich source of vitamin C, vitamin A, and fiber, enhancing the nutritional profile of the dessert. This dish is ideal for a post-workout recovery meal or as a healthy dessert option to help maintain energy levels.

CHAPTER 8
THE 31 DAY MEAL PLAN WITH EACH DAY ALTERNATE

This meal plan alternates between low-carb and high-carb days to help optimize fat loss while preserving muscle mass and supporting metabolic health. Below is a detailed menu that utilizes the recipes found in Chapters 6 (low-carb recipes) and 7 (high-carb recipes) of your book.

Day 1: Low-Carb Day

- Breakfast: Avocado and Egg Toast (Chapter 6)
- Lunch: Chicken Caesar Salad (Chapter 6)
- Dinner: Grilled Pork Chops with Herb Butter (Chapter 6)
- Snack: Cucumber Hummus Bites (Chapter 6)

Day 2: High-Carb Day

- Breakfast: Banana Oat Pancakes (Chapter 7)
- Lunch: Quinoa and Black Bean Salad (Chapter 7)
- Dinner: Teriyaki Chicken with Steamed Rice (Chapter 7)
- Snack: Banana Berry Smoothie (Chapter 7)

Day 3: Low-Carb Day

- Breakfast: Greek Yogurt and Nut Parfait (Chapter 6)
- Lunch: Turkey Spinach Salad with Avocado Dressing (Chapter 6)
- Dinner: Lemon Pepper Shrimp over Zucchini Noodles (Chapter 6)
- Snack: Almonds and Cheese (Chapter 6)

Day 4: High-Carb Day

- Breakfast: Whole Wheat Waffles (Chapter 7)
- Lunch: Sweet Potato and Black Bean Burrito (Chapter 7)
- Dinner: Pasta Primavera (Chapter 7)
- Snack: Apple with Peanut Butter (Chapter 7)

Day 5: Low-Carb Day

- Breakfast: Cheese and Spinach Omelette (Chapter 6)
- Lunch: Grilled Chicken Salad with Olive Oil Dressing (Chapter 6)
- Dinner: Beef Stir-Fry with Mixed Vegetables (Chapter 6)
- Snack: Celery Sticks with Almond Butter (Chapter 6)

Day 6: High-Carb Day

- Breakfast: Oatmeal with Fresh Berries (Chapter 7)

- Lunch: Lentil Soup with a Slice of Whole Grain Bread (Chapter 7)
- Dinner: Stir-Fried Tofu with Brown Rice (Chapter 7)
- Snack: Yogurt with Honey and Granola (Chapter 7)

Day 7: Low-Carb Day

- Breakfast: Scrambled Eggs with Spinach and Feta (Chapter 6)
- Lunch: Caesar Salad with Grilled Shrimp (Chapter 6)
- Dinner: Pan-Seared Salmon with Asparagus (Chapter 6)
- Snack: Avocado Slices Wrapped in Prosciutto (Chapter 6)

Day 8: High-Carb Day

- Breakfast: French Toast with Maple Syrup (Chapter 7)
- Lunch: Chickpea Salad with Cucumber, Tomato, and Feta (Chapter 7)
- Dinner: Quinoa Stuffed Bell Peppers (Chapter 7)
- Snack: Mixed Berries (Chapter 7)

Day 9: Low-Carb Day

- Breakfast: Avocado Smoothie (Chapter 6)
- Lunch: Broccoli and Chicken Stir Fry (Chapter 6)
- Dinner: Grilled Lamb Chops with Mint Sauce (Chapter 6)
- Snack: Cheese Cubes with Walnuts (Chapter 6)

Day 10: High-Carb Day

- Breakfast: Pancakes with Blueberries (Chapter 7)
- Lunch: Vegetable and Bean Chili (Chapter 7)
- Dinner: Baked Cod with Sweet Potato Fries (Chapter 7)
- Snack: Rice Cakes with Avocado (Chapter 7)

Day 11: Low-Carb Day

- Breakfast: Mushroom and Spinach Frittata (Chapter 6)
- Lunch: Tuna Salad with Avocado (Chapter 6)
- Dinner: Grilled Turkey Burgers with Lettuce Wraps (Chapter 6)
- Snack: Macadamia Nuts (Chapter 6)

Day 12: High-Carb Day

- Breakfast: Bagel with Cream Cheese and Tomato (Chapter 7)
- Lunch: Roasted Vegetable and Hummus Wrap (Chapter 7)
- Dinner: Chicken Paella (Chapter 7)
- Snack: Fruit Salad (Chapter 7)

Day 13: Low-Carb Day

- Breakfast: Cheese and Herb Omelette (Chapter 6)
- Lunch: Cobb Salad with Blue Cheese Dressing (Chapter 6)
- Dinner: Pork Tenderloin with Roasted Brussels Sprouts (Chapter 6)
- Snack: Greek Yogurt with Sliced Almonds (Chapter 6)

Day 14: High-Carb Day

- Breakfast: Porridge with Raisins and Brown Sugar (Chapter 7)
- Lunch: Falafel with Pita Bread and Tzatziki Sauce (Chapter 7)
- Dinner: Spaghetti with Marinara Sauce (Chapter 7)
- Snack: Popcorn (Chapter 7)

Day 15: Low-Carb Day

- Breakfast: Smoked Salmon and Cream Cheese Rolls (Chapter 6)
- Lunch: Grilled Steak Salad with Arugula and Parmesan (Chapter 6)
- Dinner: Chicken Stir-Fry with Mixed Green Vegetables (Chapter 6)
- Snack: Sliced Cucumbers with Ranch Dip (Chapter 6)

Day 16: High-Carb Day

- Breakfast: Smoothie Bowl with Oats, Banana, and Honey (Chapter 7)
- Lunch: Baked Sweet Potatoes with Black Beans and Corn (Chapter 7)
- Dinner: Thai Green Curry with Jasmine Rice (Chapter 7)
- Snack: Granola Bar (Chapter 7)

Day 17: Low-Carb Day

- Breakfast: Spinach and Goat Cheese Scramble (Chapter 6)
- Lunch: Shrimp and Avocado Salad (Chapter 6)
- Dinner: Beef and Broccoli (Chapter 6)
- Snack: Beef Jerky (Chapter 6)

Day 18: High-Carb Day

- Breakfast: French Toast with Strawberries (Chapter 7)
- Lunch: Lentil and Spinach Soup with Crusty Bread (Chapter 7)
- Dinner: Vegetarian Lasagna (Chapter 7)
- Snack: Pear Slices with Honey (Chapter 7)

Day 19: Low-Carb Day

- Breakfast: Keto Blueberry Muffins (Chapter 6)
- Lunch: Caesar Salad with Grilled Chicken (Chapter 6)
- Dinner: Seared Tuna Steaks with Olive Tapenade (Chapter 6)

- Snack: Olives and Cheese (Chapter 6)

Day 20: High-Carb Day

- Breakfast: Oatmeal with Sliced Bananas and Almonds (Chapter 7)
- Lunch: Veggie Burger with Sweet Potato Wedges (Chapter 7)
- Dinner: Shrimp Risotto (Chapter 7)
- Snack: Baked Apple with Cinnamon (Chapter 7)

Day 21: Low-Carb Day

- Breakfast: Greek Yogurt with Flaxseeds and Walnuts (Chapter 6)
- Lunch: Beef Lettuce Wraps with Sriracha Mayo (Chapter 6)
- Dinner: Grilled Chicken with Roasted Mediterranean Vegetables (Chapter 6)
- Snack: Hard-Boiled Eggs (Chapter 6)

Day 22: High-Carb Day

- Breakfast: Banana and Peanut Butter Smoothie (Chapter 7)
- Lunch: Quinoa Salad with Roasted Chickpeas (Chapter 7)
- Dinner: Baked Ziti with Ricotta and Marinara (Chapter 7)
- Snack: Trail Mix with Dried Fruit and Nuts (Chapter 7)

Day 23: Low-Carb Day

- Breakfast: Ham and Cheese Omelette (Chapter 6)
- Lunch: Chopped Salad with Grilled Salmon (Chapter 6)
- Dinner: Lamb Chops with Mint Yogurt Sauce and Steamed Green Beans (Chapter 6)
- Snack: Cucumber Slices with Guacamole (Chapter 6)

Day 24: High-Carb Day

- Breakfast: Muesli with Skim Milk and Fresh Berries (Chapter 7)
- Lunch: Turkey and Avocado Wrap with Whole Wheat Tortilla (Chapter 7)
- Dinner: Vegetarian Stir Fry with Tofu and Brown Rice (Chapter 7)
- Snack: Rice Pudding (Chapter 7)

Day 25: Low-Carb Day

- Breakfast: Cottage Cheese with Sliced Peaches (Chapter 6)
- Lunch: Grilled Portobello Mushroom Burger (No Bun) (Chapter 6)
- Dinner: Roast Beef with Cauliflower Mash (Chapter 6)
- Snack: Almond Butter Celery Sticks (Chapter 6)

Day 26: High-Carb Day

- Breakfast: Pancakes with Apple Sauce (Chapter 7)
- Lunch: Black Bean Soup with Cornbread (Chapter 7)

- Dinner: Penne Pasta with Tomato Basil Sauce (Chapter 7)
- Snack: Orange Slices (Chapter 7)

Day 27: Low-Carb Day

- Breakfast: Poached Eggs with Sautéed Spinach (Chapter 6)
- Lunch: Chicken Caesar Salad without Croutons (Chapter 6)
- Dinner: Grilled Swordfish with Lemon Butter Sauce and Asparagus (Chapter 6)
- Snack: Pepperoni Slices with Mozzarella Cheese (Chapter 6)

Day 28: High-Carb Day

- Breakfast: Oatmeal with Honey and Sliced Almonds (Chapter 7)
- Lunch: Sweet Potato and Lentil Curry with Rice (Chapter 7)
- Dinner: Chicken Enchiladas (Chapter 7)
- Snack: Yogurt with Mixed Berries (Chapter 7)

Day 29: Low-Carb Day

- Breakfast: Avocado and Egg Salad on Rye Bread (Skip bread for lower carbs) (Chapter 6)
- Lunch: Nicoise Salad with Tuna (Chapter 6)
- Dinner: Pork Tenderloin with a Side of Roasted Brussels Sprouts (Chapter 6)
- Snack: Sliced Radishes with Salt and Lemon Juice (Chapter 6)

Day 30: High-Carb Day

- Breakfast: French Toast with Berry Compote (Chapter 7)
- Lunch: Chickpea and Spinach Stew with Couscous (Chapter 7)
- Dinner: Seafood Paella (Chapter 7)
- Snack: Baked Pita Chips with Hummus (Chapter 7)

Day 31: Low-Carb Day

- Breakfast: Smoked Salmon with Cream Cheese on Cucumber Slices (Chapter 6)
- Lunch: Turkey Meatballs with Zucchini Noodles (Chapter 6)
- Dinner: Grilled Ribeye Steak with Side Salad (Chapter 6)
- Snack: Cheese Sticks (Chapter 6)

CHAPTER 9
ADVANCED PHASE OF THE 31-DAY ALTERNATING MEAL PLAN

Day 1: Low-Carb

- Breakfast: Avocado and Egg Toast (Chapter 6)
- Lunch: Chicken Caesar Salad (Chapter 6)
- Dinner: Zesty Lemon Garlic Salmon (Chapter 6)
- Snack: Cucumber Hummus Bites (Chapter 6)
- Dessert: Almond Flour Chocolate Chip Cookies (Chapter 6)

Day 2: Low-Carb

- Breakfast: Greek Yogurt and Nut Parfait (Chapter 6)
- Lunch: Beef and Broccoli (Chapter 6)
- Dinner: Grilled Chicken with Asparagus (Chapter 6)
- Snack: Cheese and Walnut Stuffed Celery (Chapter 6)
- Dessert: Peanut Butter Balls (Chapter 6)

Day 3: High-Carb

- Breakfast: Oatmeal with Fresh Berries (Chapter 7)
- Lunch: Quinoa Salad with Mixed Vegetables (Chapter 7)
- Dinner: Pasta Primavera (Chapter 7)
- Snack: Banana and Nut Butter (Chapter 7)
- Dessert: Baked Apple with Honey and Cinnamon (Chapter 7)

Day 4: High-Carb

- Breakfast: Smoothie Bowl with Mixed Fruits (Chapter 7)
- Lunch: Sweet Potato and Black Bean Burrito (Chapter 7)
- Dinner: Brown Rice and Vegetable Stir Fry (Chapter 7)
- Snack: Trail Mix (Chapter 7)
- Dessert: Mango Sorbet (Chapter 7)

Day 5: High-Carb

- Breakfast: Pancakes with Maple Syrup (Chapter 7)
- Lunch: Lentil Soup with Whole Wheat Bread (Chapter 7)
- Dinner: Baked Ziti with Marinara Sauce (Chapter 7)
- Snack: Greek Yogurt with Honey and Granola (Chapter 7)
- Dessert: Chocolate Pudding (Chapter 7)

Day 6: Low-Carb

- Breakfast: Scrambled Eggs with Spinach (Chapter 6)
- Lunch: Tuna Salad Lettuce Wraps (Chapter 6)
- Dinner: Pork Tenderloin with Cauliflower Mash (Chapter 6)
- Snack: Almonds and Cheese (Chapter 6)
- Dessert: Coconut Flour Brownies (Chapter 6)

Day 7: Low-Carb

- Breakfast: Cottage Cheese and Berries (Chapter 6)
- Lunch: Shrimp and Avocado Salad (Chapter 6)
- Dinner: Turkey Burgers with Portobello "Buns" (Chapter 6)
- Snack: Olives and Feta Cheese (Chapter 6)
- Dessert: Keto Cheesecake (Chapter 6)

Day 8: High-Carb

- Breakfast: Bagels with Cream Cheese and Smoked Salmon (Chapter 7)
- Lunch: Chickpea and Spinach Curry (Chapter 7)
- Dinner: Vegetable Lasagna (Chapter 7)
- Snack: Fruit Salad (Chapter 7)
- Dessert: Rice Pudding (Chapter 7)

Day 9: High-Carb

- Breakfast: French Toast with Berries (Chapter 7)
- Lunch: Corn Chowder with Fresh Bread (Chapter 7)
- Dinner: Couscous with Roasted Vegetables (Chapter 7)
- Snack: Apple Slices with Peanut Butter (Chapter 7)
- Dessert: Peach Cobbler (Chapter 7)

Day 10: High-Carb

- Breakfast: Blueberry Muffins (Chapter 7)
- Lunch: Tomato Basil Pasta (Chapter 7)
- Dinner: Stir-Fried Tofu with Rice (Chapter 7)
- Snack: Popcorn (Chapter 7)
- Dessert: Banana Bread (Chapter 7)

Day 11: Low-Carb

- Breakfast: Frittata with Mushrooms and Spinach (Chapter 6)
- Lunch: Grilled Salmon Salad (Chapter 6)
- Dinner: Beef Stir-Fry with Broccoli and Peppers (Chapter 6)

- Snack: Deviled Eggs (Chapter 6)
- Dessert: Dark Chocolate and Nut Clusters (Chapter 6)

Day 12: Low-Carb

- Breakfast: Protein Pancakes with Almond Butter (Chapter 6)
- Lunch: Cobb Salad (Chapter 6)
- Dinner: Chicken Thighs with Roasted Brussels Sprouts (Chapter 6)
- Snack: Avocado Slices with Lime and Salt (Chapter 6)
- Dessert: Lemon Bars (Chapter 6)

Day 13: High-Carb

- Breakfast: Porridge with Honey and Cinnamon (Chapter 7)
- Lunch: Baked Sweet Potatoes with Black Beans (Chapter 7)
- Dinner: Penne with Creamy Mushroom Sauce (Chapter 7)
- Snack: Dried Fruits and Nuts (Chapter 7)
- Dessert: Carrot Cake (Chapter 7)

Day 14: High-Carb

- Breakfast: Granola with Milk (Chapter 7)
- Lunch: Falafel Wrap with Tahini Sauce (Chapter 7)
- Dinner: Quinoa and Roasted Vegetable Salad (Chapter 7)
- Snack: Yogurt with Fruit Compote (Chapter 7)
- Dessert: Chocolate Chip Cookies (Chapter 7)

Day 15: High-Carb

- Breakfast: Pancakes with Honey and Nuts (Chapter 7)
- Lunch: Vegetable and Bean Soup with Crusty Bread (Chapter 7)
- Dinner: Spaghetti with Tomato Sauce (Chapter 7)
- Snack: Roasted Chickpeas (Chapter 7)
- Dessert: Gelato (Chapter 7)

Day 16: Low-Carb

- Breakfast: Bacon and Eggs (Chapter 6)
- Lunch: Greek Salad with Grilled Chicken (Chapter 6)
- Dinner: Stuffed Peppers with Ground Turkey (Chapter 6)
- Snack: Cheese Slices with Walnuts (Chapter 6)
- Dessert: Flourless Chocolate Cake (Chapter 6)

Day 17: Low-Carb

- Breakfast: Smoked Salmon Omelette (Chapter 6)

- Lunch: Spinach and Feta Stuffed Chicken Breast (Chapter 6)
- Dinner: Grilled Shrimp with Garlic Butter Zoodles (Chapter 6)
- Snack: Pork Rinds (Chapter 6)
- Dessert: Raspberry Mousse (Chapter 6)

Day 18: High-Carb

- Breakfast: Oatmeal with Banana and Almonds (Chapter 7)
- Lunch: Lentil and Vegetable Stew (Chapter 7)
- Dinner: Rice Pilaf with Mixed Vegetables (Chapter 7)
- Snack: Pretzels (Chapter 7)
- Dessert: Apple Pie (Chapter 7)

Day 19: High-Carb

- Breakfast: Cereal with Milk and Fruit (Chapter 7)
- Lunch: Tomato Soup and Grilled Cheese Sandwich (Chapter 7)
- Dinner: Baked Cod with Sweet Potato Fries (Chapter 7)
- Snack: Granola Bars (Chapter 7)
- Dessert: Fruit Tart (Chapter 7)

Day 20: High-Carb

- Breakfast: Waffles with Strawberry Sauce (Chapter 7)
- Lunch: Veggie Burger with Coleslaw (Chapter 7)
- Dinner: Pad Thai with Tofu (Chapter 7)
- Snack: Rice Cakes with Avocado (Chapter 7)
- Dessert: Chocolate Soufflé (Chapter 7)

Day 21: Low-Carb

- Breakfast: Keto Blueberry Muffins (Chapter 6)
- Lunch: Caesar Salad with Grilled Steak Strips (Chapter 6)
- Dinner: Lemon Herb Roasted Chicken (Chapter 6)
- Snack: Mixed Nuts (Chapter 6)
- Dessert: Cheesecake Fat Bombs (Chapter 6)

Day 22: Low-Carb

- Breakfast: Coconut Flour Pancakes (Chapter 6)
- Lunch: Avocado Tuna Salad (Chapter 6)
- Dinner: Pork Chops with Sauteed Green Beans (Chapter 6)
- Snack: Sliced Cucumbers with Cream Cheese (Chapter 6)
- Dessert: Chocolate Avocado Pudding (Chapter 6)

Day 23: High-Carb

- Breakfast: Bagel with Peanut Butter and Jelly (Chapter 7)
- Lunch: Black Bean Soup with Cornbread (Chapter 7)
- Dinner: Vegetarian Chili with Rice (Chapter 7)
- Snack: Baked Potato Chips (Chapter 7)
- Dessert: Brownies (Chapter 7)

Day 24: High-Carb

- Breakfast: Smoothie with Banana, Berries, and Oats (Chapter 7)
- Lunch: Pita Sandwich with Falafel (Chapter 7)
- Dinner: Stir-Fry with Noodles and Vegetables (Chapter 7)
- Snack: Popcorn with Parmesan (Chapter 7)
- Dessert: Panna Cotta with Berry Compote (Chapter 7)

Day 25: High-Carb

- Breakfast: Yogurt with Granola and Honey (Chapter 7)
- Lunch: Roasted Beet and Goat Cheese Salad (Chapter 7)
- Dinner: Pizza with a Variety of Toppings (Chapter 7)
- Snack: Fresh Fruit Salad (Chapter 7)
- Dessert: Lemon Sorbet (Chapter 7)

Day 26: Low-Carb

- Breakfast: Ham and Cheese Omelette (Chapter 6)
- Lunch: Broccoli and Cheddar Soup (Chapter 6)
- Dinner: Grilled Tilapia with Lemon Butter (Chapter 6)
- Snack: Beef Jerky (Chapter 6)
- Dessert: Keto Ice Cream (Chapter 6)

Day 27: Low-Carb

- Breakfast: Bulletproof Coffee (Chapter 6)
- Lunch: Caprese Salad with Balsamic Reduction (Chapter 6)
- Dinner: Beef Stroganoff with Mushroom (Chapter 6)
- Snack: Celery Sticks with Almond Butter (Chapter 6)
- Dessert: Strawberry Cheesecake (Chapter 6)

Day 28: High-Carb

- Breakfast: French Crepes with Jam (Chapter 7)
- Lunch: Minestrone Soup (Chapter 7)
- Dinner: Moroccan Couscous with Roasted Vegetables (Chapter 7)

- Snack: Honey Roasted Nuts (Chapter 7)
- Dessert: Tiramisu (Chapter 7)

Day 29: High-Carb

- Breakfast: Bagels with Cream Cheese and Fresh Berries (Chapter 7)
- Lunch: Quiche Lorraine with a Side Salad (Chapter 7)
- Dinner: Vegetable Paella (Chapter 7)
- Snack: Baked Sweet Potato Wedges (Chapter 7)
- Dessert: Fruit Sorbet (Chapter 7)

Day 30: High-Carb

- Breakfast: Porridge with Raisins and Brown Sugar (Chapter 7)
- Lunch: Chickpea Salad Sandwich (Chapter 7)
- Dinner: Spaghetti with Marinara Sauce and Meatballs (Chapter 7)
- Snack: Fruit Smoothie (Chapter 7)
- Dessert: Chocolate Lava Cake (Chapter 7)

Day 31: Low-Carb

- Breakfast: Keto Bagels with Cream Cheese (Chapter 6)
- Lunch: Chicken Caesar Wrap (using low-carb tortillas) (Chapter 6)
- Dinner: Filet Mignon with Garlic Butter Mushrooms (Chapter 6)
- Snack: Hard-Boiled Eggs (Chapter 6)
- Dessert: Pumpkin Spice Mousse (Chapter 6)

CONCLUSION

Glossary of Key Terms and Definitions

When embarking on any new nutrition plan, it helps to clarify key terminologies to fully grasp concepts and implement them effectively. Below are succinct definitions of vital carb cycling vocabulary:

- **Macronutrients** - The three main nutrients that provide calories: carbohydrates, protein, and fat. Tracking macros involves calculating ideal intake of each based on goals.

- **Carbohydrates** - One of the three macronutrients; found in grains, starchy veggies, fruits, dairy, and legumes. Carbs break down into glucose for energy.

- **High carb days** - Days on a carb cycling plan when you consume more carbohydrates, typically for energizing hard workouts or refueling post-exercise. High days range from 200-300+ grams of carbs.

- **Low carb days** - Days on a carb cycling plan when you restrict carbohydrates to 50-150 grams to burn stored fat and enter ketosis. Low carb days alternate with high-carb days.

- **Ketosis** - A metabolic state where your body burns fat for fuel instead of carbs. Ketosis is triggered by very low carb intake, fasting, or strenuous exercise.

- **Net carbs** - Total carbs minus fiber equals net carbs. Fiber doesn't raise blood sugar, so it's excluded from carb counts. Prioritize high fiber carbs with lower net carbs.

- **Protein** - Muscle-building macronutrient crucial for repair, hormones, and enzyme function. Whey, eggs, meats, fish, dairy, and legumes contain protein. Shoot for 0.7-1 gram per pound of body weight daily.

- **Fat** - Macronutrient that supports hormone function, nutrient absorption, and metabolism. Healthy fats like olive oil, nuts, seeds, avocado, and oily fish provide essential fatty acids and satiety. Most diets get 30-40% calories from fats.

- **Calories** - Units of energy obtained from carbohydrates, protein, and fat in food and drink. A caloric deficit from reduced carb/calorie intake spurs fat loss on lower carb days.

- **Glycogen** - The stored form of glucose derived from carbohydrates, housed primarily in the muscles and liver. Glycogen provides quick energy for intense exercise.

- **Insulin** - Hormone made by the pancreas that allows cells to use glucose from carbs for energy by transporting it from the bloodstream. Low carb diets aim to control insulin.

- **Gluconeogenesis** - The body's process of manufacturing glucose from non-carb sources like protein or fat; happens in ketosis or fasting when carbs are scarce. Allows brain function using ketones from fat.

- **Macronutrient Cycling** - Alternating higher and lower amounts of carbohydrates and fats from day to day on a structured schedule to reap different benefits of each.

- **Refuel Days** - Higher carb days following intense training sessions to restore glycogen and repair depleted muscles. Typically, 1.5-2 grams of carbs per pound of bodyweight.

- **Isocaloric** - When calories stay consistent each day despite macro differences. Isocaloric carb cycling aims for a steady daily calorie target.

- **Non-Isocaloric** - Varying calories and macros together, so low carb days induce a deficit and high carb days a surplus. More dramatic fat loss potential.

- **Clean Eating** - Emphasizing whole, minimally processed foods like produce, lean proteins, legumes, nuts/seeds and healthy fats while limiting refined grains, sweets, and fried foods.

- **Whole Foods** - Foods close to their natural, unprocessed state, like vegetables, fruits, eggs, and raw nuts. Higher in nutrition without additives.

EXTRA CONTENTS

Full Macro Calculator

The "Full Macro Calculator" is a must-have tool to easily customize your diet plan, helping you accurately calculate the macronutrients appropriate for your health and fitness goals.

Food Calorie Calculator

"Food Calorie Calculator," offers users the ability to accurately track daily caloric intake, making it easier to manage a balanced diet geared toward specific weight loss or fitness maintenance goals.

Meal Planner and Shopping List

The bonus 'Meal Planner and Shopping List (printable)' included in the 'Carb Cycling Cookbook for Beginners' is essential for planning your meals weekly in an organized manner. This tool helps you compile an accurate shopping list, ensuring that you always have the ingredients you need to effectively adhere to your carb cycling plan, allowing you to save money and reduce waste.

Pressure and Glycemia Calculator

The "Pressure and Glycemia Calculator" is a valuable resource for those who wish to monitor their blood pressure and blood glucose levels

Audiobook

The included audiobook is perfect for those who prefer an aural approach to learning, offering the convenience of exploring diet strategies and tasty recipes without having to stare at a screen or page.

EBOOK: Illustrated Chair Yoga Exercises

The bonus "Illustrated Chair Yoga Exercises" is a useful visual guide for anyone who wants to integrate gentle and accessible yoga practices into their daily routine, perfect for increasing flexibility and reducing stress without leaving the chair.

EBOOK: Carb Cycling Cookbook for Beginners with IMAGE

The bonus "EBOOK: Carb Cycling Cookbook for Beginners with IMAGE" enhances the reading experience with color photographs of each recipe, making every dish not only visually appealing but also easy to replicate at home, perfect for those new to carb cycling.

Merry Lott

Scan the QR CODE Below

Printed in Great Britain
by Amazon

58016179R00071